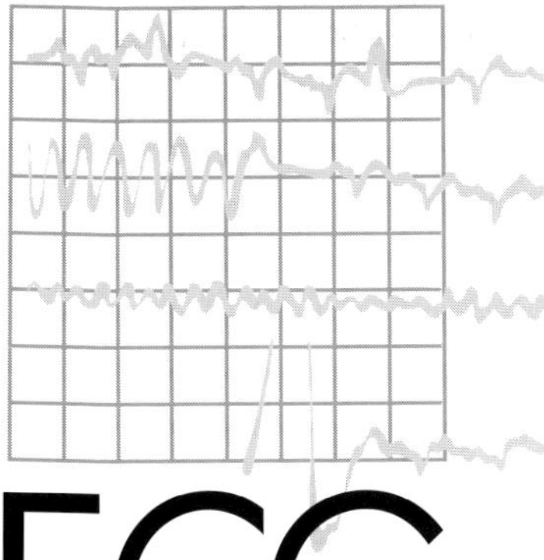

SECOND EDITION

150 ECG PROBLEMS

Commissioning Editor: Laurence Hunter
Project Development Manager: Lynn Watt and Helius
Project Manager: Nancy Arnott
Designer: Erik Bigland and Helius
Illustrator: Helius and Chartwell Illustrators
Illustration Manager: Bruce Hogarth

SECOND EDITION

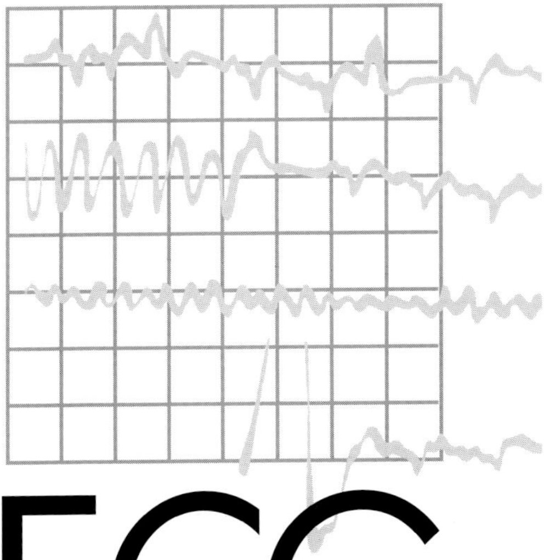

150 ECG PROBLEMS

John R. Hampton DM MA DPhil FRCP FFPM FESC

Emeritus Professor of Cardiology
University of Nottingham
Nottingham
UK

CHURCHILL LIVINGSTONE

EDINBURGH LONDON NEW YORK OXFORD PHILADELPHIA
ST LOUIS SYDNEY TORONTO 2003

CHURCHILL LIVINGSTONE An imprint of Elsevier Science Limited

First edition 1997
Second edition 2003
Reprinted 2003

Standard edition ISBN 0 443 072485
International edition ISBN 0 443 072493

British Library Cataloguing in Publication Data
A catalogue record for this book is available from the British Library

Library of Congress Cataloging in Publication Data
A catalog record for this book is available from the Library of Congress

Note

Medical knowledge is constantly changing. Standard safety precautions must be followed, but as new research and clinical experience broaden our knowledge, changes in treatment and drug therapy may become necessary or appropriate. Readers are advised to check the most current product information provided by the manufacturer of each drug to be administered to verify the recommended dose, the method and duration of administration, and contraindications. It is the responsibility of the practitioner, relying on experience and knowledge of the patient, to determine dosages and the best treatment for each individual patient. Neither the Publisher nor the author assumes any liability for any injury and/or damage to persons or property arising from this publication.

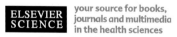

The publisher's policy is to use **paper manufactured from sustainable forests**

Printed in China
P/02

Preface

Learning about ECG interpretation from books such as *The ECG Made Easy* or *The ECG in Practice* is fine so far as it goes, but it never goes far enough. As with most of medicine, there is no substitute for experience, and to make the best use of the ECG there is no substitute for reviewing large numbers of them. ECGs need to be seen in the context of the patient from whom they were recorded. You have to learn to appreciate the variations both of normality and of the patterns associated with different diseases, and to think about how the ECG can help patient management.

Although no book can substitute for practical experience, *150 ECG Problems* goes a stage nearer the clinical world than books that simply aim to teach ECG interpretation. It presents 150 clinical problems in the shape of simple case histories, together with the relevant ECG. It invites the reader to interpret the ECG in the light of the clinical evidence provided, and to decide on a course of action before looking at the answer. Having seen the answers, the reader may feel the need for more information, so each one is cross-referenced to *The ECG Made Easy* or *The ECG in Practice*.

The ECGs in *150 ECG Problems* range from the simple to the complex. About one-third of the problems are of a standard that a medical student should be able to cope with, and will be answered correctly by anyone who has read *The ECG Made Easy*. A house officer, specialist nurse or paramedic should get another third right, and will certainly be able to do so if they have read *The ECG in Practice*. The remainder should challenge the MRCP candidate.

As a very rough guide to the level of difficulty, each answer is given one, two or three stars (see the summary box of each answer): one star represents the easiest records, and three stars the most difficult.

The ECGs are arranged in random order, not in order of difficulty: this is to maintain interest and to challenge the reader to attempt an interpretation before looking at the star rating. This is, after all, the real-life situation: one never knows which patient will be easy and which will be difficult to diagnose or treat.

150 ECG Problems is the successor to *100 ECG Problems*, published in 1997. The popularity of the latter has encouraged me to include more examples of common abnormalities and also some problems for which there was previously no space. I hope the reader will find *150 ECG Problems* an entertaining and an easy way to learn and revise.

John R. Hampton
Nottingham

The symbols **ME** and **IP** denote cross-references to useful information in the books *The ECG Made Easy*, 6th edn, and *The ECG in Practice*, 4th edn, respectively (written by Professor Hampton and published by Elsevier Science).

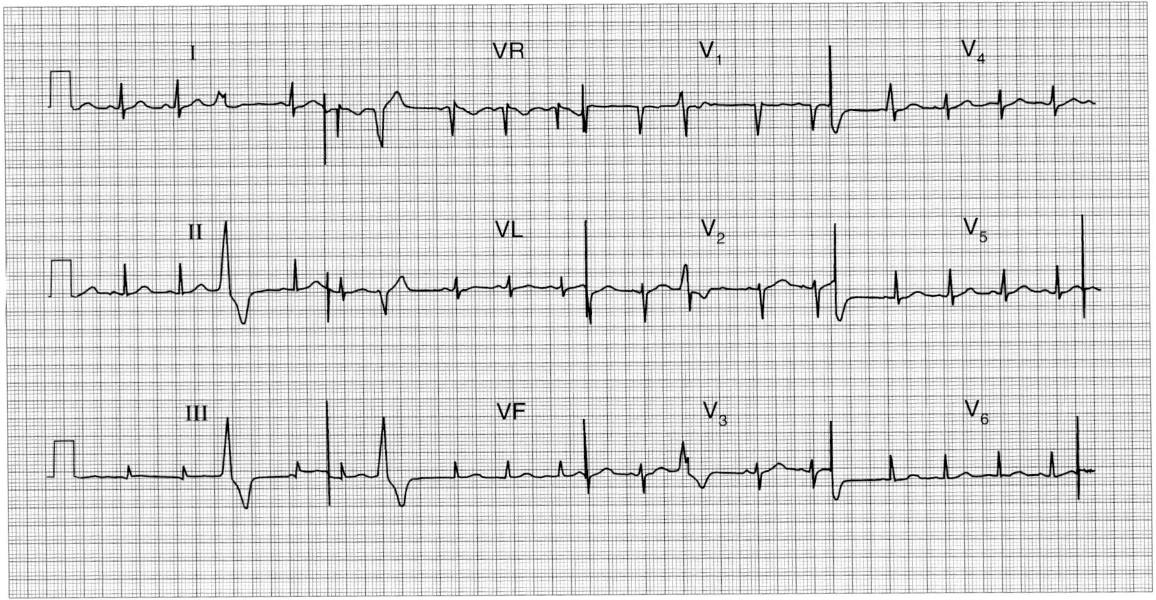

ECG 1 This ECG was recorded from a 25-year-old pregnant woman who complained of an irregular heart beat. Auscultation revealed a soft systolic murmur but her heart was otherwise normal. What does the ECG show and what would you do?

ANSWER 1

The ECG shows:

- Sinus rhythm
- Ventricular extrasystoles
- Normal axis
- Normal QRS complexes and T waves

Clinical interpretation

The extrasystoles are fairly frequent but the ECG is otherwise normal. Ventricular extrasystoles are very common in pregnancy, and systolic murmurs are almost universal. Her heart is almost certainly normal.

What to do

Remember that anaemia is a common cause of a systolic murmur. Doubts about the significance of the murmur can be resolved by echocardiography, but this need not be performed in every pregnant woman – it is best reserved for the investigation of apparently important murmurs that persist after delivery. The patient should be reassured and the extrasystoles left untreated.

Summary ★
Sinus rhythm with ventricular extrasystoles.

ME See p. 64
IP See p. 155

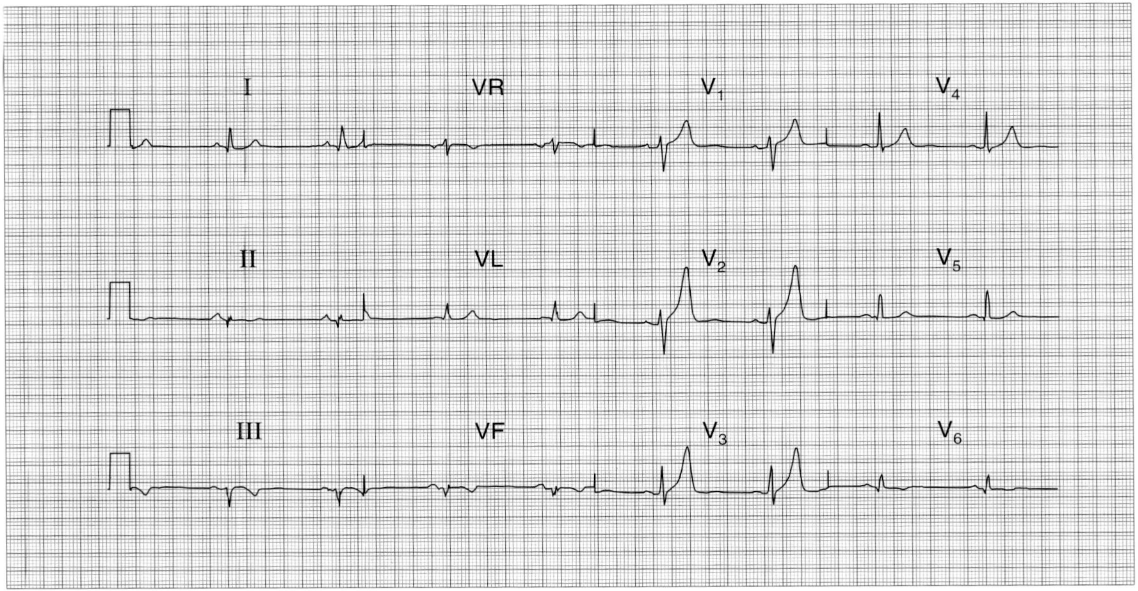

ECG 2 A 60-year-old man was seen as an out-patient, complaining of rather vague central chest pain on exertion. He had never had pain at rest. What does this ECG show and what would you do next?

ANSWER 2

The ECG shows:

- Sinus rhythm
- Normal axis
- Small Q waves in leads II, III, VF
- Biphasic T waves in leads II, V_6; inverted T waves in leads III, VF
- Markedly peaked T waves in leads V_1–V_2

Clinical interpretation

The Q waves in the inferior leads, together with inverted T waves, point to an old inferior myocardial infarction. While symmetrically peaked T waves in the anterior leads can be due to hyperkalaemia, or to ischaemia, they are frequently a normal variant.

What to do

The patient seems to have had a myocardial infarction at some point in the past, and by implication his vague chest pain may be due to cardiac ischaemia. Attention must be paid to risk factors (smoking, blood pressure, plasma cholesterol), and he probably needs long-term treatment with aspirin and a statin. An exercise test will be the best way of deciding whether he has coronary disease that merits angiography.

Summary ★

Old inferior myocardial infarction.

ME See p. 103

IP See p. 238

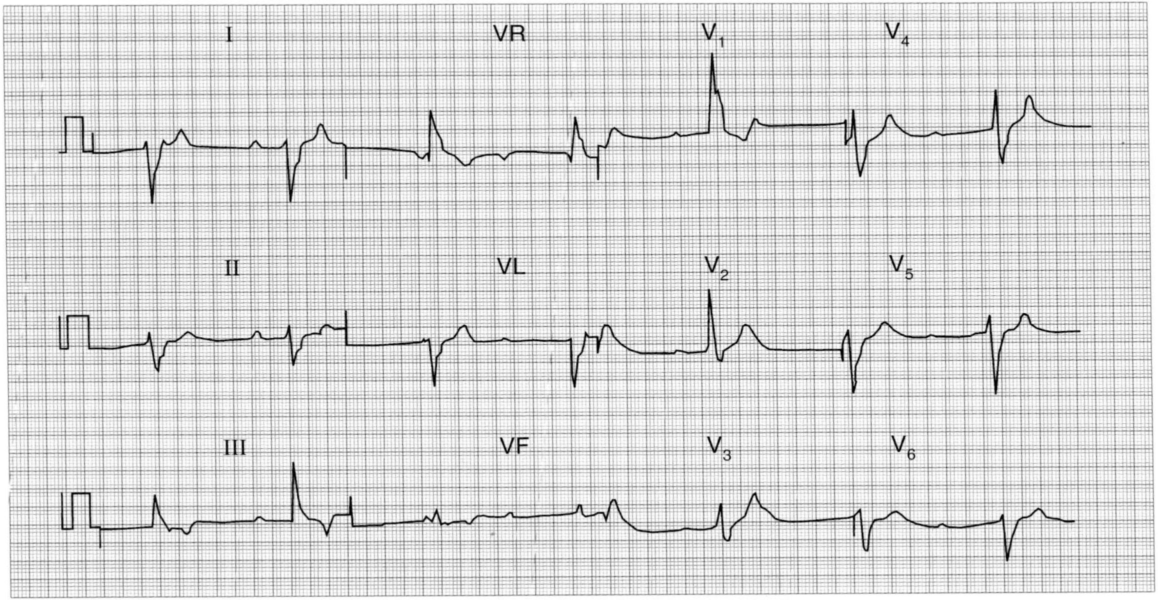

ECG 3 An 80-year-old woman, who had previously had a few attacks of dizziness, fell and broke her hip. She was found to have a slow pulse, and this is her ECG. The surgeons want to operate as soon as possible but the anaesthetist is unhappy. What does the ECG show and what should be done?

ANSWER 3

The ECG shows:

- Complete heart block
- Ventricular rate 45/min

Clinical interpretation

In complete heart block there is no relationship between the P waves (here with a rate of 70/min) and the QRS complexes. The ventricular 'escape' rhythm has wide QRS complexes and abnormal T waves. No further interpretation of the ECG is possible.

What to do

In the absence of a history suggesting a myocardial infarction, this woman almost certainly has chronic heart block: the fall may or may not have been due to a Stokes–Adams attack. She needs a permanent pacemaker, ideally immediately to save the morbidity of first temporary, and then permanent, pacemaker insertion. If permanent pacing is not possible immediately, a temporary pacemaker will be needed preoperatively.

Summary ★
Complete (third degree) heart block.

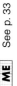

ME See p. 33

IP See p. 213

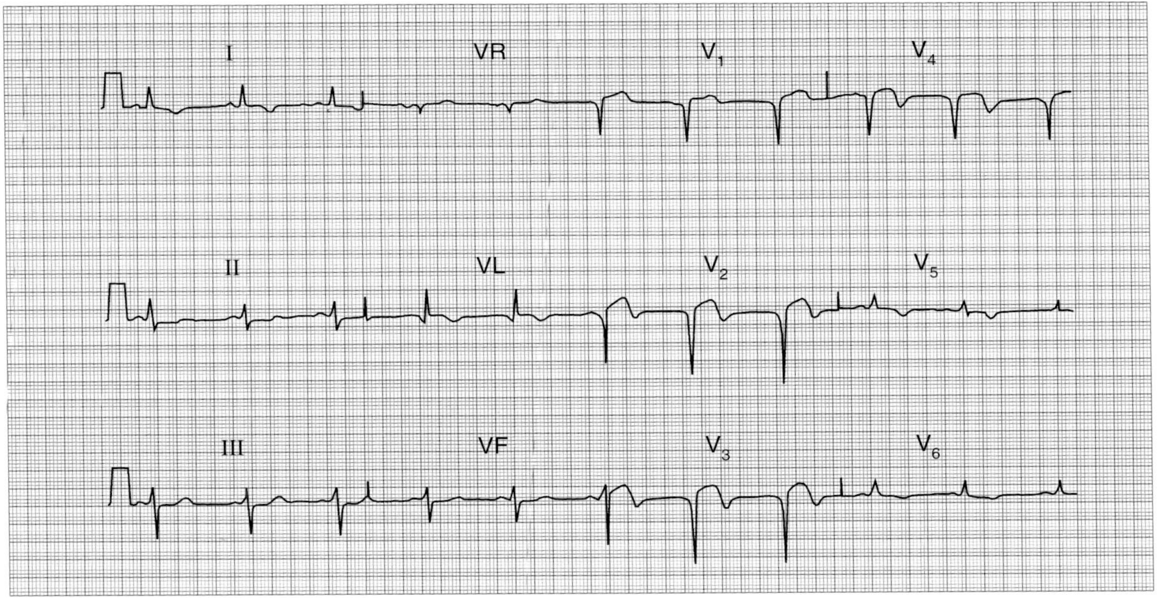

ECG 4 A 50-year-old man is seen in the A & E department with severe central chest pain which has been present for 18 h. What does this ECG show and what would you do?

ANSWER 4

The ECG shows:

- Sinus rhythm
- Normal axis
- Q waves in leads V_2–V_4
- Raised ST segments in leads V_2–V_4
- Inverted T waves in leads I, VL, V_2–V_6

Clinical interpretation

This is a classic acute anterior myocardial infarction.

What to do

More than 18 h have elapsed since the onset of pain, so this patient is outside the conventional limit for thrombolysis. Nevertheless, if he is still in pain and still looks unwell, thrombolytic treatment should be given unless there are good reasons not to do so. In any case he should be given pain relief and aspirin, and must be admitted to hospital for observation.

Summary ★
Acute anterior myocardial infarction.

ME See p. 96

IP See p. 239

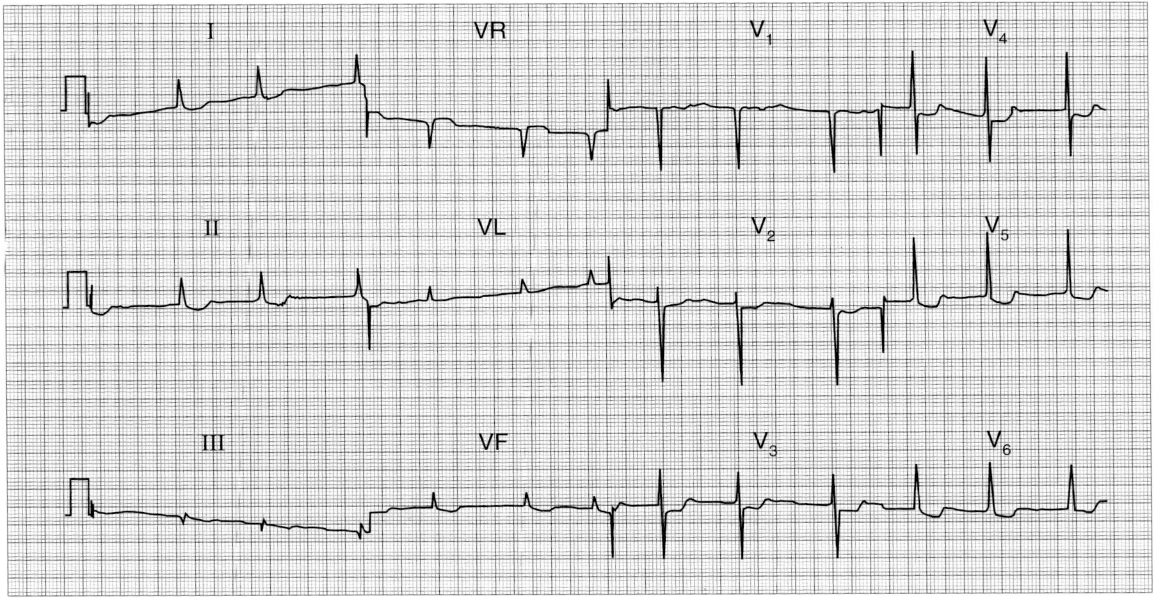

ECG 5 This ECG was recorded from a 60-year-old woman with rheumatic heart disease. She had been in heart failure, but this had been treated and she was no longer breathless. What does the ECG show and what question might you ask her?

ANSWER 5

The ECG shows:

- Atrial fibrillation with a ventricular rate of 60–65/min
- Normal axis
- Normal QRS complexes
- Prominent U wave in lead V_2
- Downward-sloping ST segments, best seen in leads V_5–V_6

Clinical interpretation

The downward-sloping ST segments (the 'reverse tick') indicate that digoxin has been given. The ventricular rate seems well-controlled. The prominent U waves in lead V_2 could indicate hypokalaemia.

What to do

Ask the patient about her appetite: the earliest symptom of digoxin toxicity is appetite loss, followed by nausea and vomiting. If the patient is being treated with diuretics, check the serum potassium level – a low potassium level potentiates the effects of digoxin. If in doubt, the serum digoxin level is easily measured.

Summary ★★
Atrial fibrillation with digoxin effect.

ME See pp. 78 and 107

IP See pp. 367 and 373

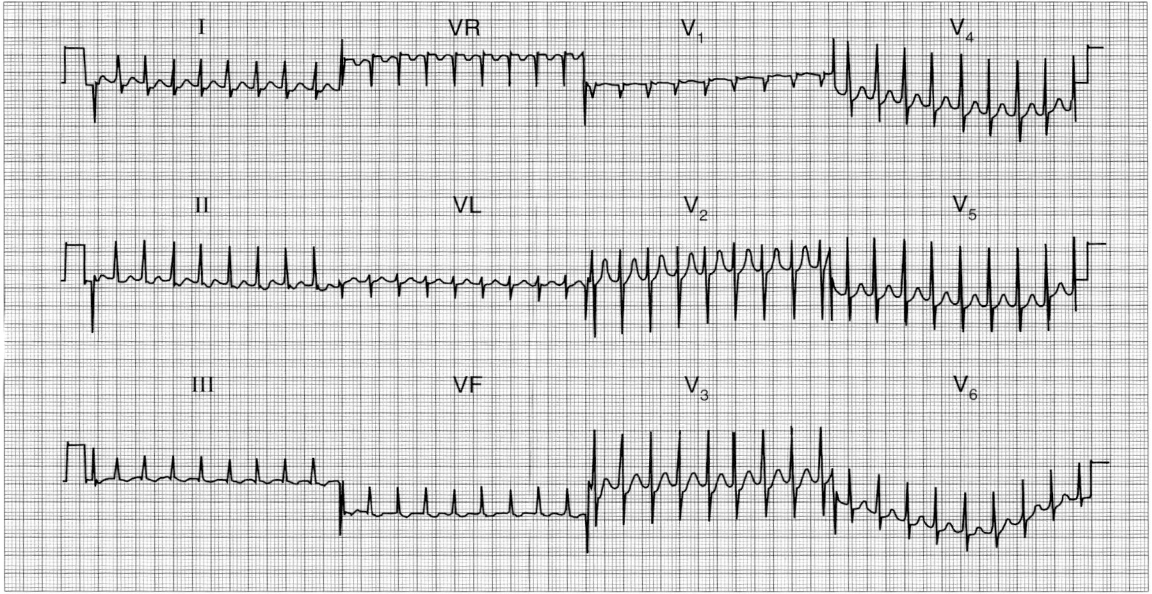

ECG 6 A 26-year-old woman, who has complained of palpitations in the past, is admitted via the A & E department with palpitations. What does the ECG show and what should you do?

ANSWER 6

The ECG shows:

- Narrow-complex tachycardia, rate about 200/min
- No P waves visible
- Normal axis
- Regular QRS complexes
- Normal QRS complexes, ST segments and T waves

Clinical interpretation

This is a supraventricular tachycardia, and since no P waves are visible this is a junctional, or atrioventricular nodal, tachycardia.

What to do

Junctional tachycardia is the commonest form of paroxysmal tachycardia in young people, and presumably explains her previous episodes of palpitations. Attacks of junctional tachycardia may be terminated by any of the manoeuvres that lead to vagal stimulation – Valsalva's manoeuvre, carotid sinus pressure, or immersion of the face in cold water. If these are unsuccessful, intravenous adenosine should be given by bolus injection. Adenosine has a very short half-life, but can cause flushing and occasionally asthma. If adenosine proves unsuccessful, verapamil 5–10 mg given by bolus injection will usually restore sinus rhythm. Otherwise, DC cardioversion is indicated.

Summary ★
Junctional (atrioventricular nodal re-entry) tachycardia.

ME See p. 72
IP See p. 159

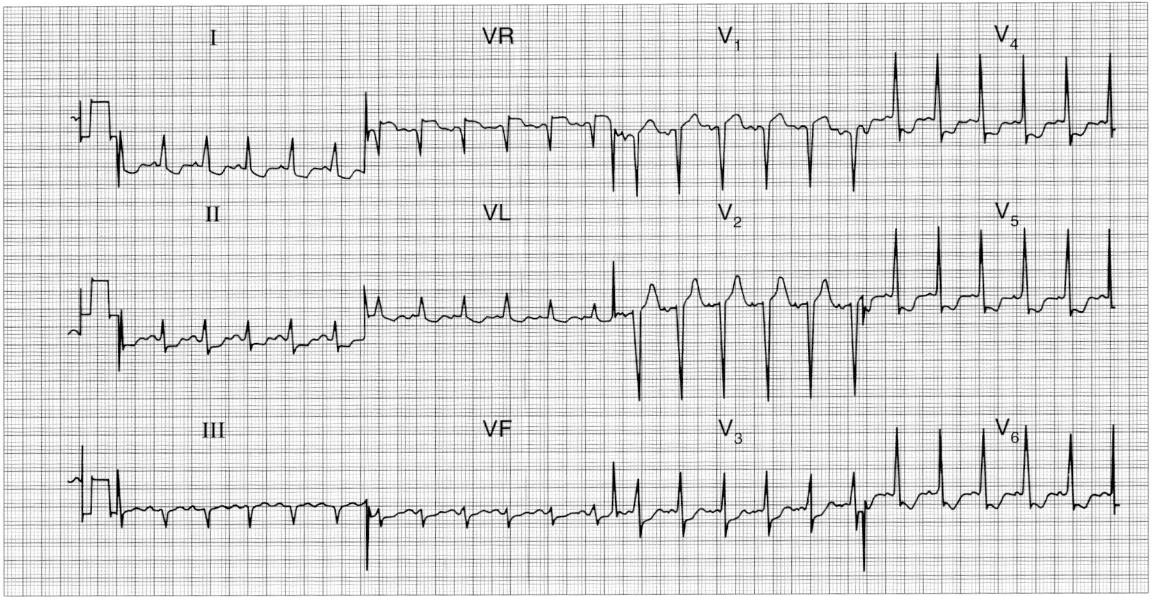

ECG 7 This ECG was recorded in the A & E department from a 55-year-old man who had had chest pain at rest for 6 h. There were no abnormal physical findings. What does the trace show, and how would you manage him?

ANSWER 7

The ECG shows:

- Sinus rhythm
- Normal axis
- Normal QRS complexes
- ST segment depression – horizontal in leads V_3–V_4, downward-sloping in leads I, VL, V_5–V_6

Clinical interpretation

This ECG shows anterior and lateral ischaemia without evidence of infarction. Taken with the clinical history, the diagnosis is clearly 'unstable' angina.

What to do

There is no evidence of any benefit from thrombolysis. The patient should be given aspirin and intravenous heparin and nitrates. At the time the record was taken, he had a sinus tachycardia (at a rate of about 130/min) and if this does not settle quickly, intravenous beta-blockade help.

Summary ★
Anterolateral ischaemia.

ME See p. 102
IP See p. 267

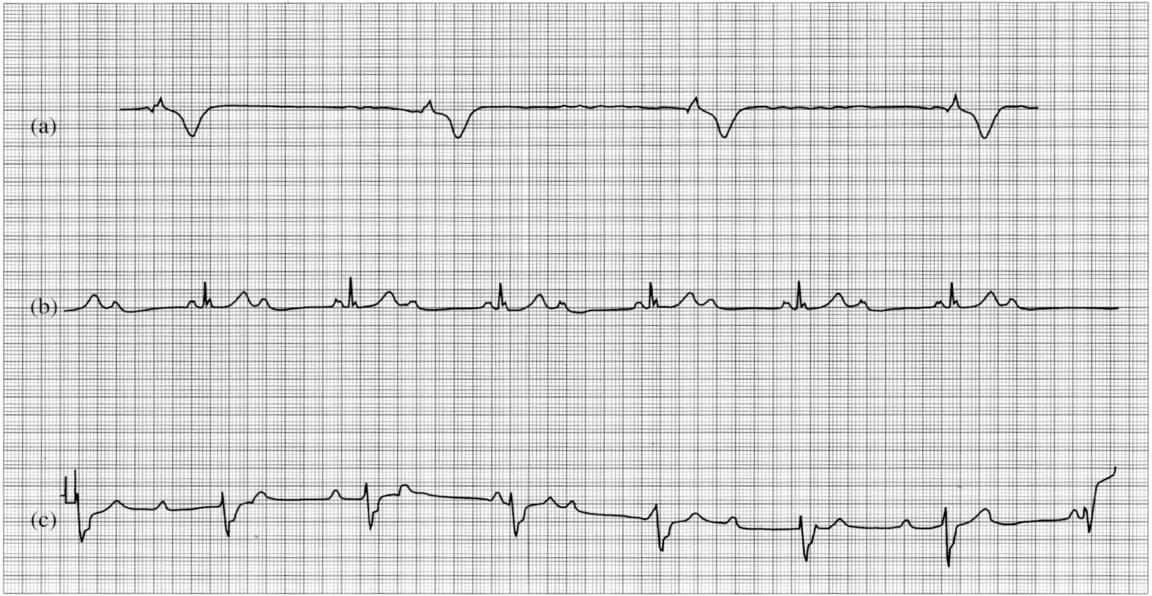

ECG 8 These three rhythm strips (all lead II) came from the ECGs of three different patients. They were all in their eighties, and all complained of breathlessness. What other symptoms might they have had, what diagnoses would you consider, and what treatment is possible?

ANSWER 8

The ECGs show:

(a) No P waves can be seen but the baseline is irregular; the QRS complexes are broad, regular, and slow. This is atrial fibrillation with complete block.
(b) In the conducted beats the PR interval is constant, so this is sinus rhythm with second degree (2:1) block. The second small deflection after the R wave is not a P wave, but is part of the QRS complex.
(c) There is no fixed relationship between the P waves and the QRS complexes, so this is complete (third degree) heart block.

Clinical interpretation

Single ECG leads can only be used to identify the rhythm, and further interpretation is unreliable.

What to do

All the patients are probably suffering the effects of their bradycardia; additional symptoms might be angina, dizziness, and collapse (Stokes–Adams attacks). In each case the likely diagnosis is idiopathic fibrosis of the conducting system, but almost all cardiac conditions can be associated with heart block – rheumatic disease, ischaemia, cardiomyopathy, trauma, metastases and so on. In the elderly, heart block is often associated with a calcified aortic valve. Whatever their age, such patients benefit from a permanent pacemaker.

Summary ★★

(a) Atrial fibrillation and complete block.
(b) Second degree (2:1) block.
(c) Complete (third degree) block.

ME See p. 30

IP See p. 199

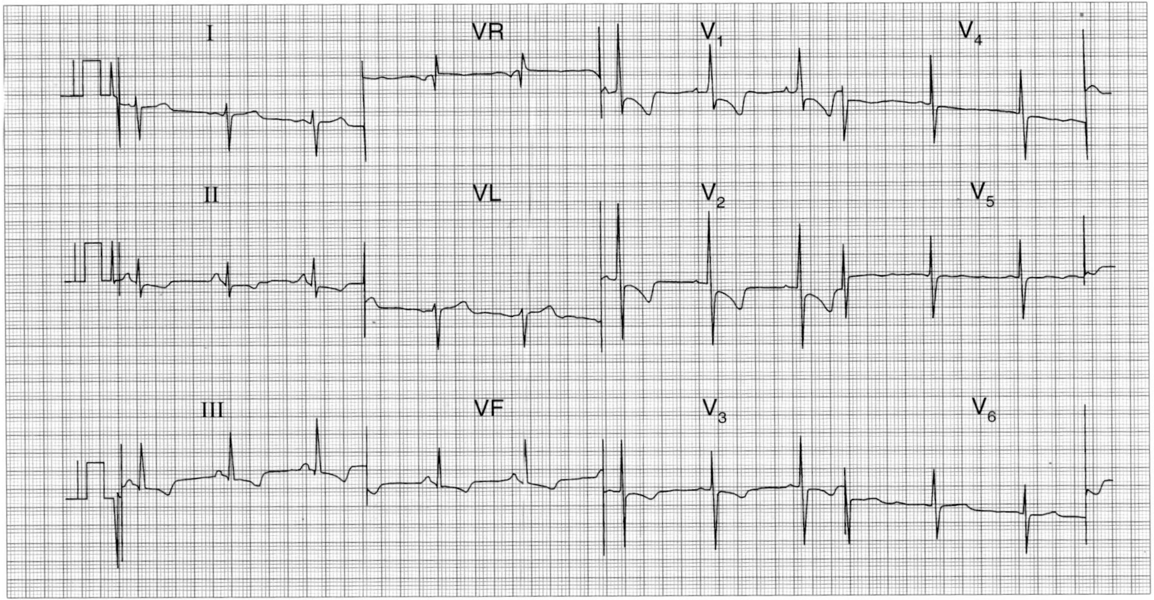

ECG 9 A 40-year-old woman is referred to the out-patient department because of increasing breathlessness. What does this ECG show, what physical signs might you expect, and what might be the underlying problem? What might you do?

ANSWER 9

The ECG shows:

- Sinus rhythm
- Peaked P waves, best seen in lead II
- Right axis deviation
- Dominant R waves in lead V_1
- Deep S waves in lead V_6
- Inverted T waves in leads II, III, VF, V_1–V_3

Clinical interpretation

This combination of right axis deviation, dominant R waves in lead V_1 and inverted T waves spreading from the right side of the heart, is classical of severe right ventricular hypertrophy. Right ventricular hypertrophy can result from congenital heart disease, or from pulmonary hypertension secondary to mitral valve disease, lung disease, or pulmonary embolism. The physical signs of right hypertrophy are a left parasternal heave and a displaced but diffuse apex beat. There may be a loud pulmonary second sound. The jugular venous pressure may be elevated and a 'flicking A' wave in the jugular venous pulse is characteristic.

What to do

The two main causes of pulmonary hypertension of this degree in a 40-year-old woman are recurrent pulmonary emboli, and primary pulmonary hypertension. Clinically, it is difficult to differentiate between the two, but a lung scan may help. In either case anticoagulants are indicated. In fact, this patient had primary pulmonary hypertension and eventually needed heart and lung transplantation.

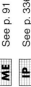

Summary ★
Severe right ventricular hypertrophy.

ME See p. 91

IP See p. 336

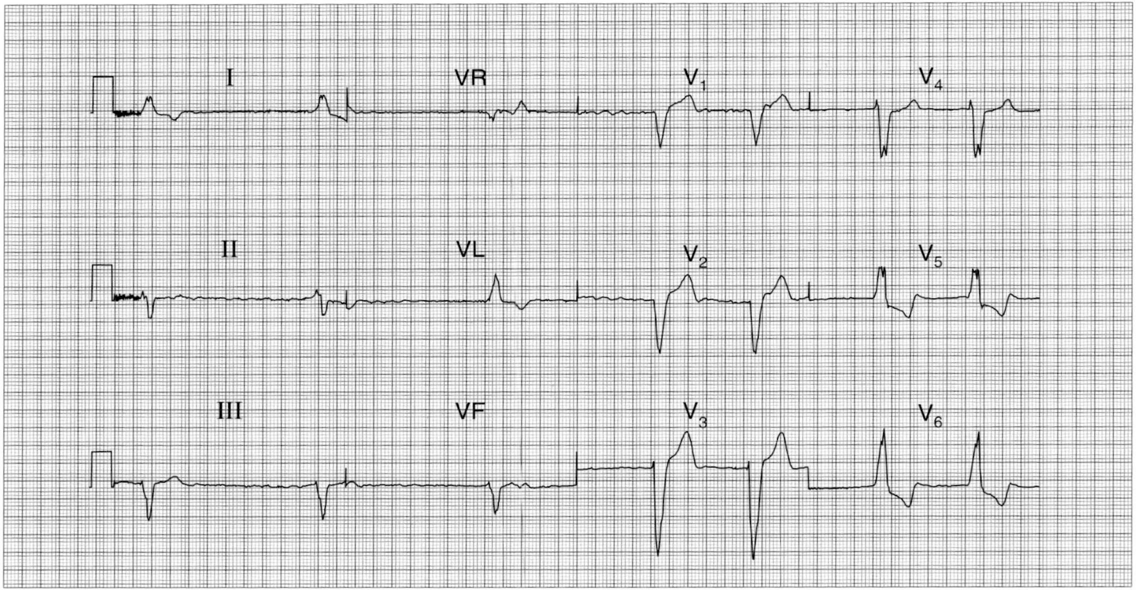

ECG 10 This ECG was recorded from an 80-year-old man who complained of breathlessness and ankle swelling which had become slowly worse over the preceding few months. He had had no chest pain and was on no treatment. He had a slow pulse, and signs of heart failure. What does the ECG show and how would you manage him?

ANSWER 10

The ECG shows:

- Atrial fibrillation with a ventricular rate of about 40/min
- Left axis
- Left bundle branch block

Clinical interpretation

When an ECG shows left bundle branch block, no further interpretation is usually possible. Here there is atrial fibrillation, and the ventricular response is very slow, suggesting that there is conduction delay in the His bundle as well as the left bundle branch.

What to do

It is always important to establish the cause of heart failure. In this patient the slow ventricular rate may be at least part of the problem. The most important causes of left bundle branch block are ischaemia, aortic stenosis and cardiomyopathy. In this patient an echocardiogram will show whether he has significant valve disease and how impaired left ventricular function is. In the absence of pain, coronary angiography is probably not indicated. The heart failure needs to be treated with diuretics and an angiotensin-converting enzyme inhibitor, but digoxin must be avoided as it may slow the ventricular response still further. He almost certainly needs a permanent pacemaker.

Summary ★

Atrial fibrillation and left bundle branch block.

ME See pp. 36 and 78

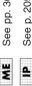

IP See p. 209

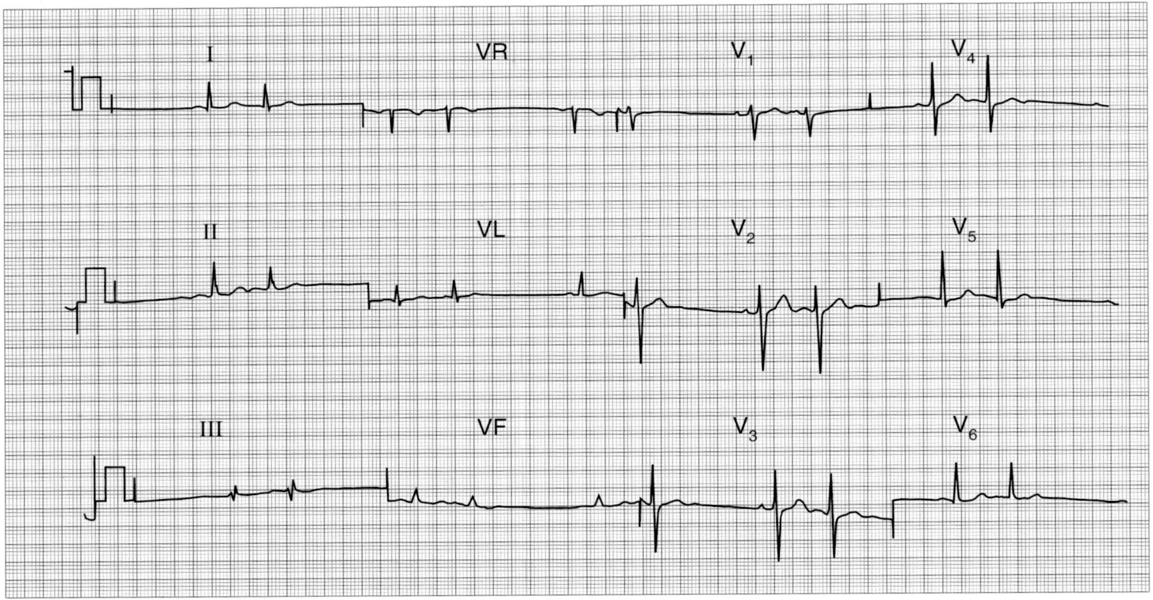

ECG 11 This ECG came from a 40-year-old woman who complained of palpitations, which were present when the recording was made. What abnormality does it show?

ANSWER 11

The ECG shows:

- Sinus rhythm
- Atrial extrasystoles, identified by early beats with broad and abnormal P waves (best seen in leads V_2 and V_3)
- Extrasystoles are followed by a 'compensatory pause'
- Normal axis
- There is an RSR pattern in lead III, but the QRS complex is narrow
- The ST segments and T waves are normal

Clinical interpretation

Since the patient had her symptoms at the time of the recording, we can be confident that the ECG findings explain her symptoms. Atrial extrasystoles, like junctional (atrioventricular nodal) extrasystoles, are not a manifestation of cardiac disease.

What to do

Provided there is nothing else in the history or examination suggesting cardiac disease, the patient can be assured that her heart is normal.

Summary ★
Sinus rhythm with atrial extrasystoles.

ME See p. 62

IP See p. 150

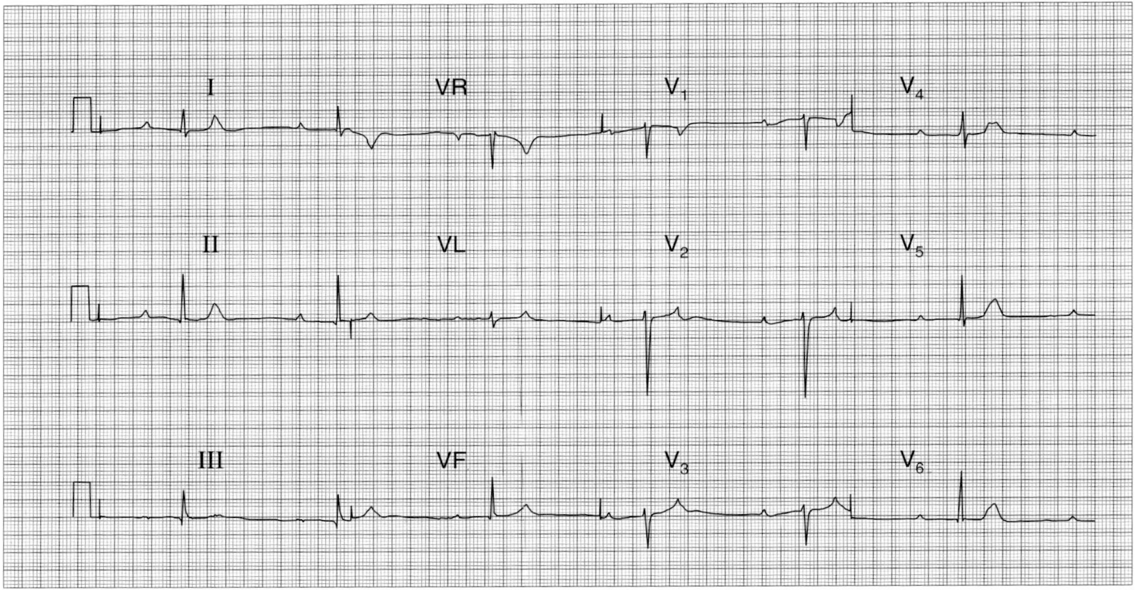

ECG 12 A 90-year-old woman is admitted to hospital after a fall resulting in a fractured hip. On questioning she admits to breathless and 'dizzy turns' for several months. This is her preoperative ECG. What does it show and what would you do?

ANSWER 12

The ECG shows:

- Second degree (2:1) heart block
- Prolonged PR interval (440 ms) in the conducted beats
- Ventricular rate about 40/min
- Normal QRS complexes and T waves

Clinical interpretation

Although the slow ventricular response raises the possibility of complete heart block, the fact that the PR interval is constant (albeit prolonged) shows that this is actually second degree block. The non-conducted P waves are not easy to see, but the clue lies in the abnormally shaped T waves in the anterior leads. Second degree block explains why the QRS complexes are narrow and the T waves are normal.

What to do

Since this woman has been breathless and dizzy for some time, and since there is nothing in the history or on the ECG to suggest an acute infarction, it is unlikely that this conduction disturbance is new. She therefore needs a permanent pacemaker: the only problem is to decide whether the urgent hip surgery should be covered with a temporary pacemaker – ideally she would be saved that procedure and a permanent system implanted immediately.

Summary ★
Second degree (2:1) heart block.

ME See p. 31

IP See p. 212

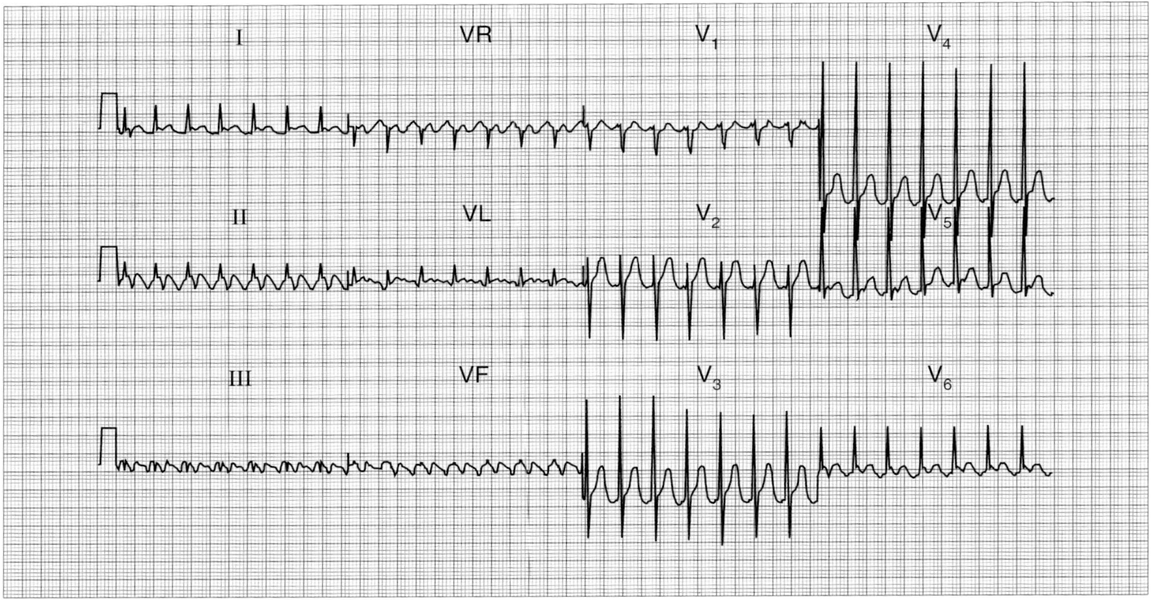

ECG 13 This ECG was recorded from a 40-year-old man who was admitted to hospital as an emergency with the sudden onset of symptoms and signs of severe left ventricular failure. What does it show and what would you do?

ANSWER 13

The ECG shows:

- Atrial flutter with 2:1 block (best seen in leads II, VR, VF)
- Normal axis
- Normal QRS complexes and T waves

Clinical interpretation

The sudden onset of atrial flutter presumably explains the heart failure. There is nothing on the ECG to suggest a cause for the arrhythmia.

What to do

When an arrhythmia causes severe heart failure, immediate treatment is more important than establishing the underlying diagnosis. Carotid sinus pressure and adenosine may increase the degree of block, but are unlikely to convert the heart to sinus rhythm. It is worth trying intravenous flecainide, but a patient with severely compromised circulation is best promptly treated with DC cardioversion.

Summary ★

Atrial flutter with 2:1 block.

ME See p. 68

IP See p. 160

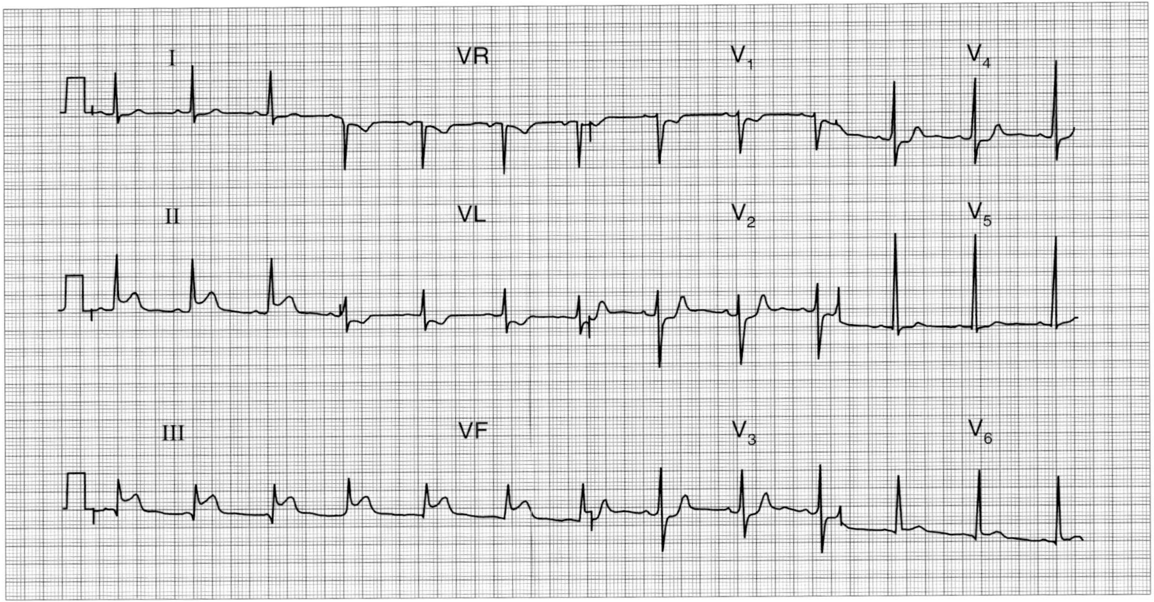

ECG 14 A 50-year-old man is admitted to hospital as an emergency, having had chest pain characteristic of a myocardial infarction for 4 h. Apart from the features associated with pain there are no abnormal physical findings. What does this ECG show and what would you do?

ANSWER 14

The ECG shows:

- Sinus rhythm
- Normal axis
- Small Q waves in lead III but not elsewhere
- Elevated ST segments in leads II, III, VF, with upright T waves
- T wave inversion in lead VL
- Suggestion of ST segment depression in leads V_2–V_3

Clinical interpretation

A classic ECG of an acute inferior myocardial infarction, with lead VL indicating ischaemia. The rate of development of Q waves is very variable: compare this record with ECG 32, which came from a patient with a similar duration of symptoms.

What to do

Pain relief must take priority. In the absence of contraindications (i.e. risk of bleeding from any important site), the patient should be given aspirin and then a thrombolytic agent.

Summary ★
Acute inferior myocardial infarction.

ME See p. 96
IP See p. 237

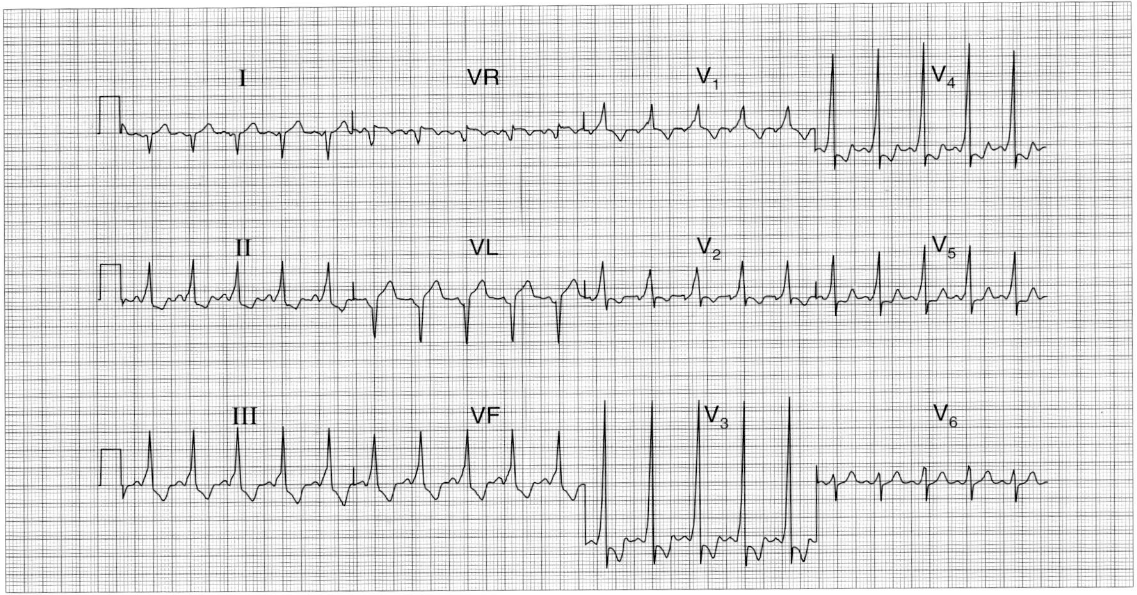

ECG 15 A 20-year-old student complains of palpitations. Attacks occur about once per year. They start suddenly, his heart feels very fast and regular, and he quickly feels breathless and faint. The attacks stop suddenly after a few minutes. There are no abnormalities on examination, and this is his ECG. What would you do?

ANSWER 15

The ECG shows:

- Sinus rhythm
- Right axis
- Short PR interval (112 ms)
- QRS complexes a little wide (124 ms)
- Slurred upstroke of QRS (delta wave)
- Dominant R wave in lead V_1
- Widespread T wave inversion

Clinical interpretation

This is a classical Wolff–Parkinson–White syndrome. The resemblance to the ECG of right ventricular hypertrophy is because this is type A, with a left-sided accessory pathway. The ECG changes of right axis, the dominant R wave in lead V_1, and the T wave changes have no further significance.

What to do

The patient gives a clear story of a paroxysmal tachycardia, and during attacks the circulation is clearly compromised because he feels dizzy. The attacks are infrequent so there is little point in ambulatory ECG recording. He needs immediate referral to an electrophysiologist for ablation of the aberrant conducting pathway.

Summary ★

Wolff–Parkinson–White syndrome type A.

ME See p. 81

IP See pp. 126 and 198

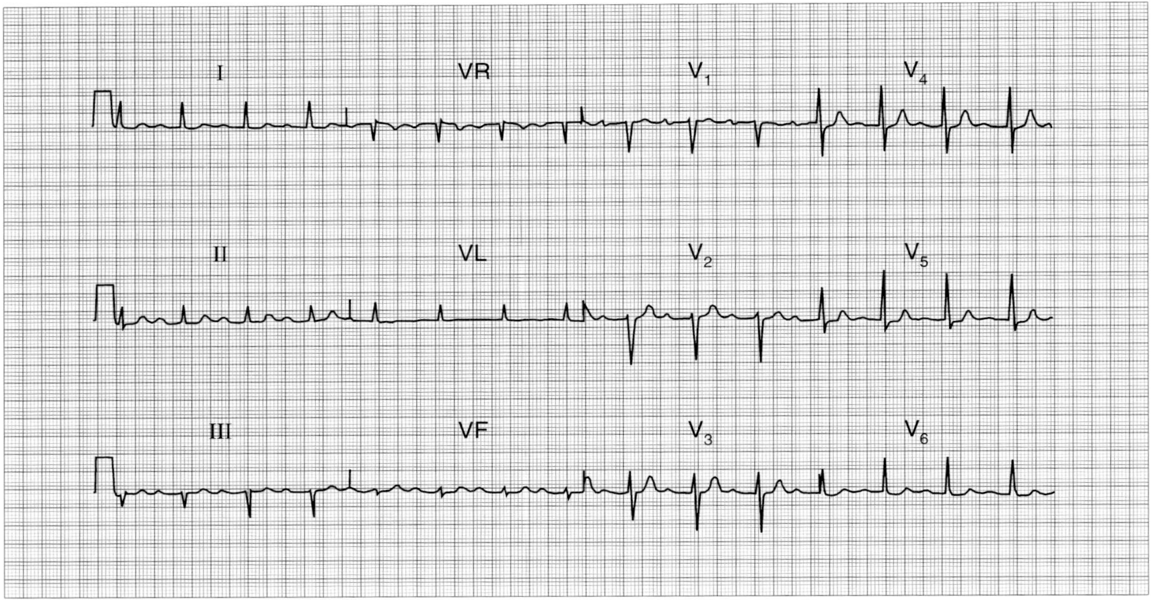

ECG 16 This ECG was recorded from a 75-year-old woman who complained of attacks of dizziness. It shows one abnormality: what is its significance?

ANSWER 16

The ECG shows:

- Sinus rhythm
- Prolonged PR interval of 280 ms (best seen in leads V_1, V_2)
- Normal axis
- Normal QRS complexes
- Normal ST segments and T waves

Clinical interpretation

Sinus rhythm with first degree block.

What to do

First degree block does not cause any haemodynamic impairment, and by itself is of little significance. However, when a patient has symptoms which might be due to a bradycardia (in this case dizziness), there may be episodes of second or third degree block, or possibly Stokes–Adams attacks, associated with a slow ventricular rate. The appropriate action is therefore to request a 24 h ECG tape-recording invthe hope that the patient will have one of her dizzy turns while wearing it. It would then be possible to see whether or not the dizziness was associated with a change in heart rhythm. First degree block itself is not an indication for permanent pacing or for any other intervention.

Summary ★★

Sinus rhythm with first degree block.

ME See p. 30

IP See p. 137

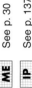

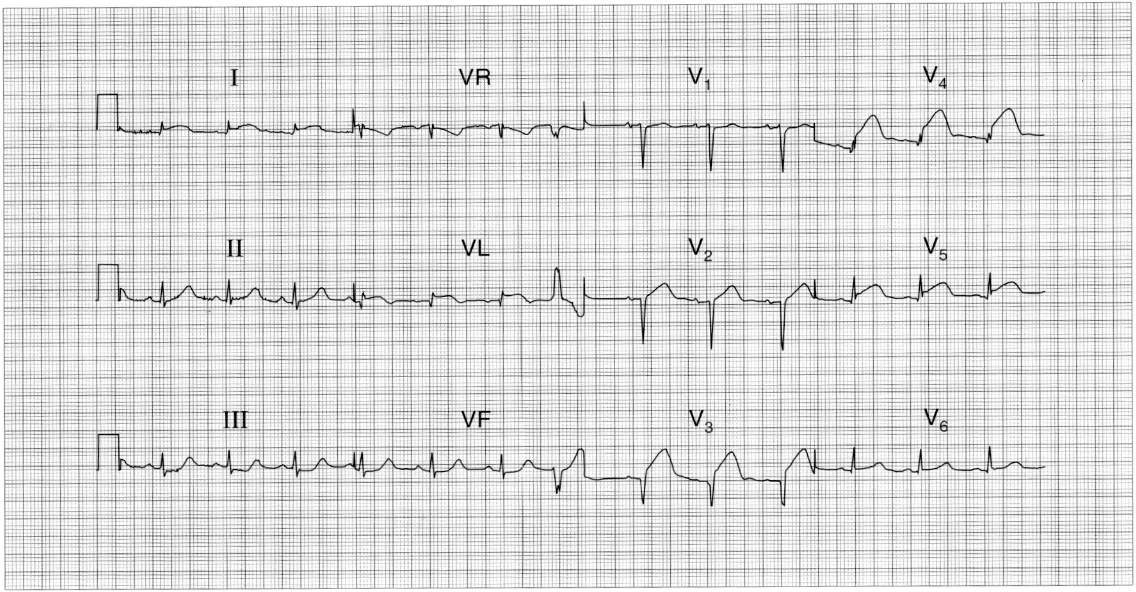

ECG 17 This ECG was recorded in the A & E department from a 60-year-old man who had had severe central chest pain for 1 h. What does it show and what would you do?

ANSWER 17

The ECG shows:

- Sinus rhythm
- One ventricular extrasystole
- Normal axis
- Q waves in leads V_2–V_3; small Q waves in leads VL, V_4
- Raised ST segments in leads I, VL, V_3–V_5

Clinical interpretation

Acute anterolateral myocardial infarction is indicated. Although a Q wave is well developed in lead V_3, the changes are entirely consistent with the story of pain for 1 h.

What to do

This patient needs pain relief with diamorphine. The ECG shows raised ST segments of more than 2 mm in several leads, so he needs immediate thrombolysis once any excess risk of bleeding has been excluded. This treatment should not be delayed by waiting for a chest X-ray or any other investigations, and should be commenced in the A & E department before transfer to the coronary care unit. Ventricular extrasystoles do not need treating.

Summary ★

Acute anterolateral myocardial infarction.

ME See p. 96

IP See p. 242

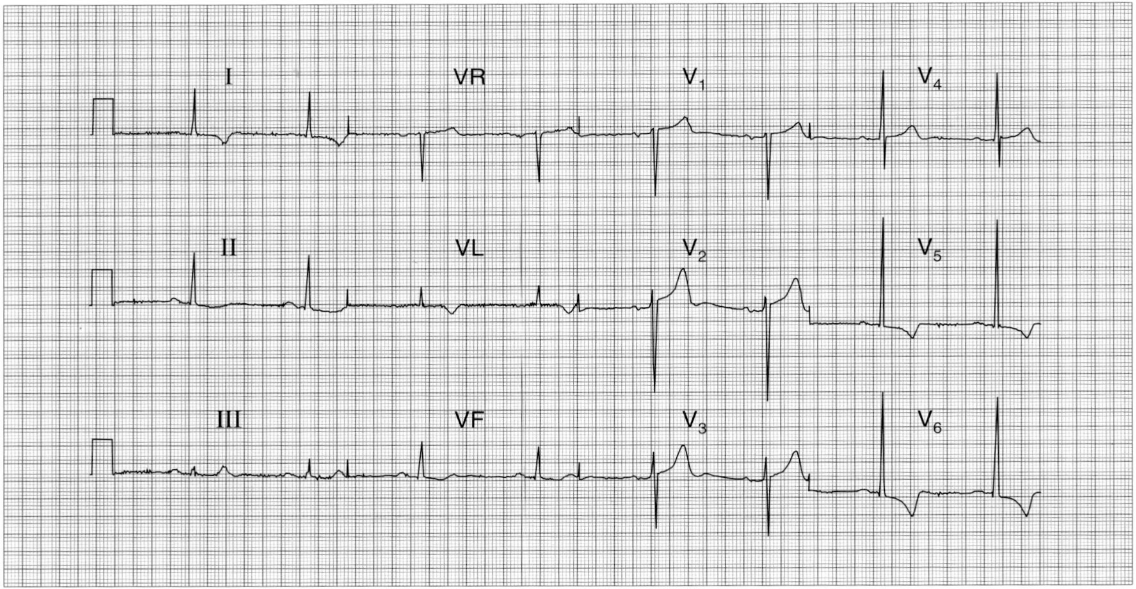

ECG 18 A 70-year-old retired orthopaedic surgeon telephones to say that he always gets dizzy playing golf. You find that he has a systolic heart murmur, and this is his ECG. What is the diagnosis and what do you do next?

ANSWER 18

The ECG shows:

- Sinus rhythm, rate 48/min
- Normal axis
- QRS duration normal, but the R wave height in lead V_5 is 30 mm, and the S wave depth in lead V_2 is 25 mm
- Inverted T waves in leads I, VL, V_5–V_6

Clinical interpretation
This is the classical ECG appearance of left ventricular hypertrophy.

What to do
The combination of dizziness on exercise, a systolic murmur, and evidence of left ventricular hypertrophy suggests significant aortic stenosis. The next step is an echocardiogram: in this patient it showed a gradient across the aortic valve of 140 mmHg, indicating severe stenosis. He needed an urgent aortic valve replacement.

Summary ★
Left ventricular hypertrophy.

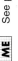

ME See p. 93
IP See p. 117

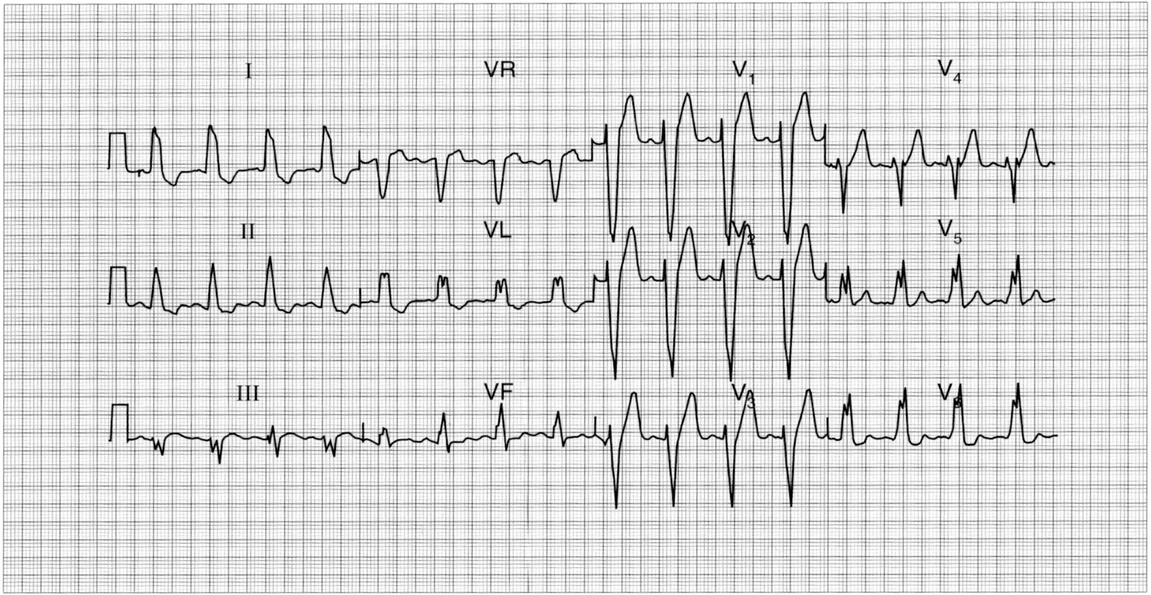

ECG 19 A 75-year-old woman complaining of central chest discomfort on climbing hills, together with dizziness; on one occasion she had 'fainted' while climbing stairs. What abnormality does this ECG show and what physical signs would you look for?

ANSWER 19

The ECG shows:

- Sinus rhythm
- Broad QRS complexes (140 ms)
- 'M' pattern in lead V_6
- Inverted T waves in leads I, VL, V_6

Clinical interpretation

This is a characteristic pattern of left bundle branch block. The ECG cannot be interpreted further.

What to do

A patient who has chest pain that could be angina, and who has dizziness and syncope on exertion, probably has severe aortic stenosis and this was the case with this woman. Clinically she had a slow rising pulse, a blood pressure of 100/80, and a slightly enlarged heart. There was a loud ejection systolic murmur, best heard at the upper right sternal edge and radiating to both carotids. The diagnosis was confirmed by an echocardiogram, which showed a gradient across the aortic valve of about 100 mmHg. A cardiac catheter was necessary to exclude coronary disease and she then had an aortic valve replacement and made a complete recovery.

Summary ★
Sinus rhythm with left bundle branch block.

ME See p. 39

IP See p. 117

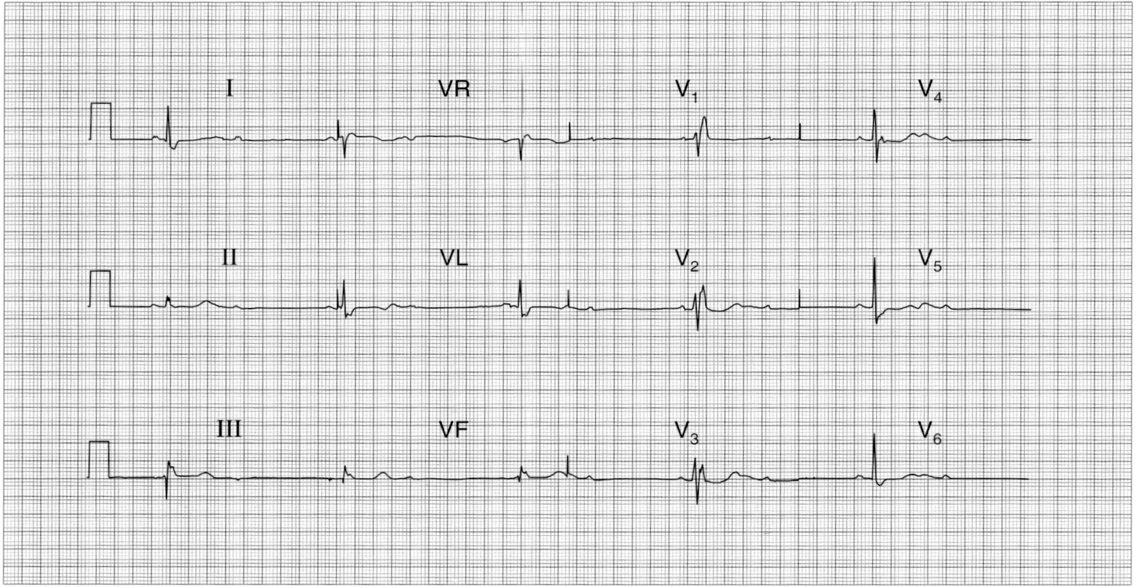

ECG 20 A 70-year-old man is seen in the clinic because of breathlessness, which began over a few days 3 months ago. This is his ECG: what does it show and what treatment is needed?

ANSWER 20

The ECG shows:

- Sinus rhythm
- Second degree (2:1) heart block (most obvious in lead V_3)
- Ventricular rate 30/min
- Normal PR interval in the conducted beats
- Normal axis
- QRS duration prolonged (160 ms)
- RSR pattern in leads V_1–V_3 and a wide S wave in lead V_6
- Prominent U wave in leads V_3–V_6

Clinical interpretation

This patient has second degree block and right bundle branch block, so he clearly has extensive conduction tissue disease.

What to do

The slow heart rate is probably the cause of his heart failure, and he needs a permanent pacemaker. The story suggests that the onset of heart failure was not associated with chest pain, so the underlying disease is probably fibrosis of the conducting system rather than ischaemia. He needs an echocardiogram and treatment with an angiotensin-converting enzyme inhibitor if there is evidence of left ventricular dysfunction.

Summary ★★
Second degree atrioventricular block and right bundle branch block.

ME See pp. 31 and 37

IP See p. 140

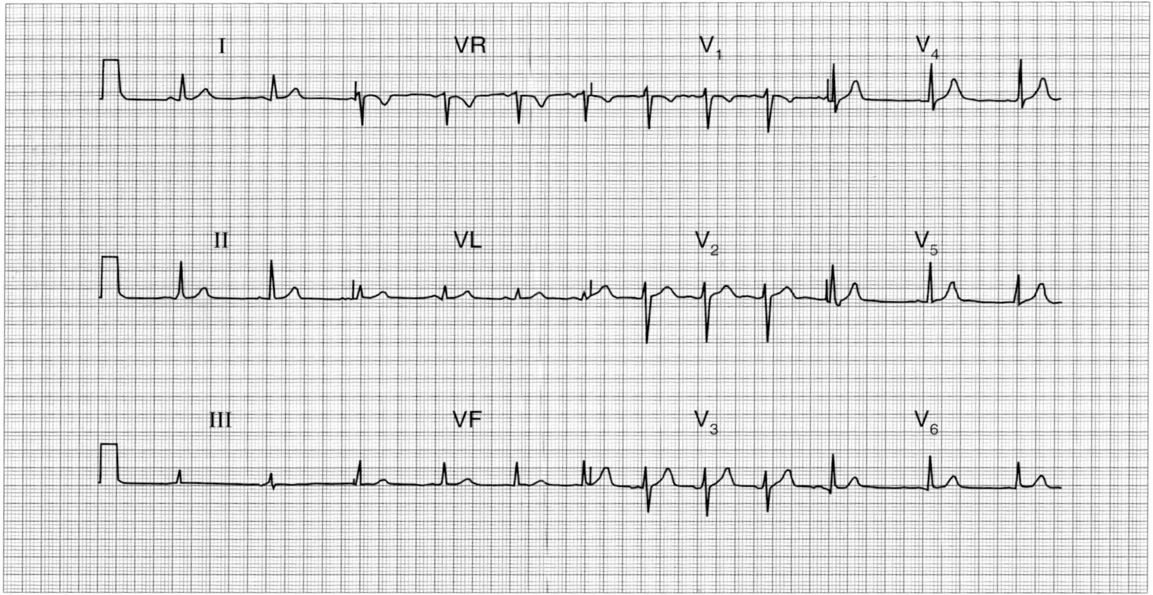

ECG 21 This ECG was recorded from a medical student during a practical class. What does it show?

ANSWER 21

The ECG shows:

- Sinus rhythm
- Sinus arrhythmia
- Normal axis
- Normal QRS complexes
- Normal ST segments and T waves

Clinical interpretation

This is a perfectly normal ECG. There is a beat-to-beat variation in the interval between QRS complexes, with the heart rate speeding up and slowing down. Comparison of the rate recorded in leads V_1, V_2 and V_3 with that recorded in leads V_4, V_5 and V_6 may give a false impression of a change of rhythm. This variation in heart rate relates to respiration and is called sinus arrhythmia, which is normal in young people. Sinus arrhythmia can be distinguished from atrial extrasystoles because in sinus arrhythmia the morphology of the P waves is unchanged.

What to do

Nothing!

Summary ★

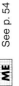

Normal ECG with sinus arrhythmia.

ME See p. 54

IP See p. 51

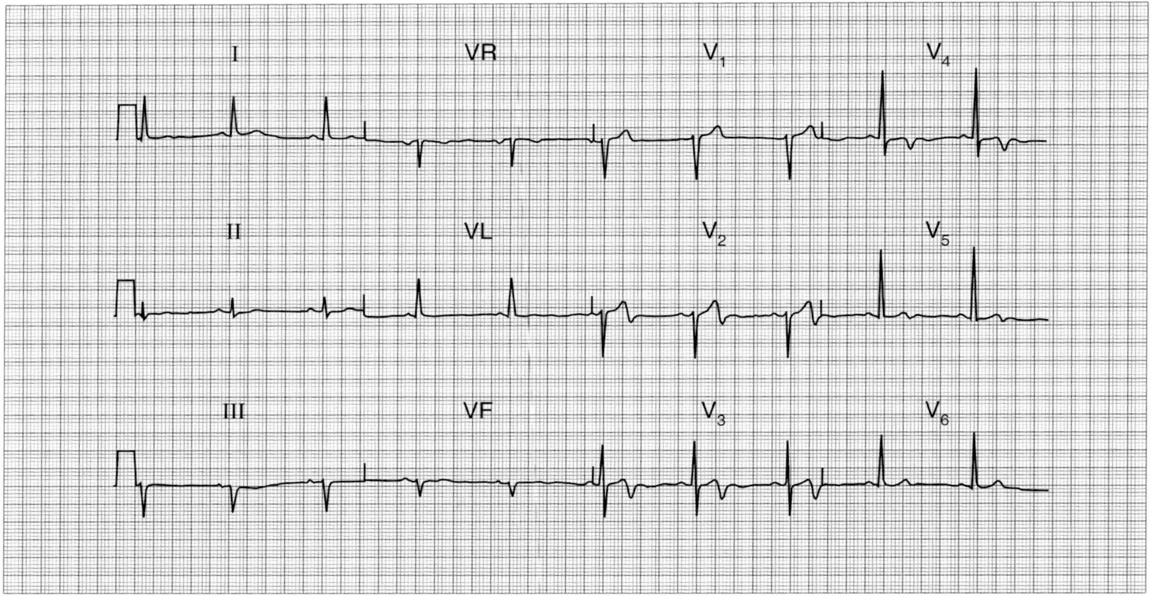

ECG 22 This ECG was recorded from a 48-year-old man who had had severe central chest pain for 1 h. What does it show and what would you do?

ANSWER 22

The ECG shows:

- Sinus rhythm
- Normal axis
- Normal QRS complexes
- Biphasic T waves in leads V_2, V_3, V_5
- Inverted T waves in lead V_4

Clinical interpretation

This is a classic acute anterior non-Q wave infarction.

What to do

This ECG does not meet the conventional criteria for thrombolysis, which are raised ST segments or new left bundle branch block. The immediate outlook is good but the patient should be monitored and the ECG repeated after an hour to see if ST segment elevation is appearing.

Summary ★
Acute anterior non-Q wave myocardial infarction.

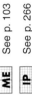

ME See p. 103

IP See p. 266

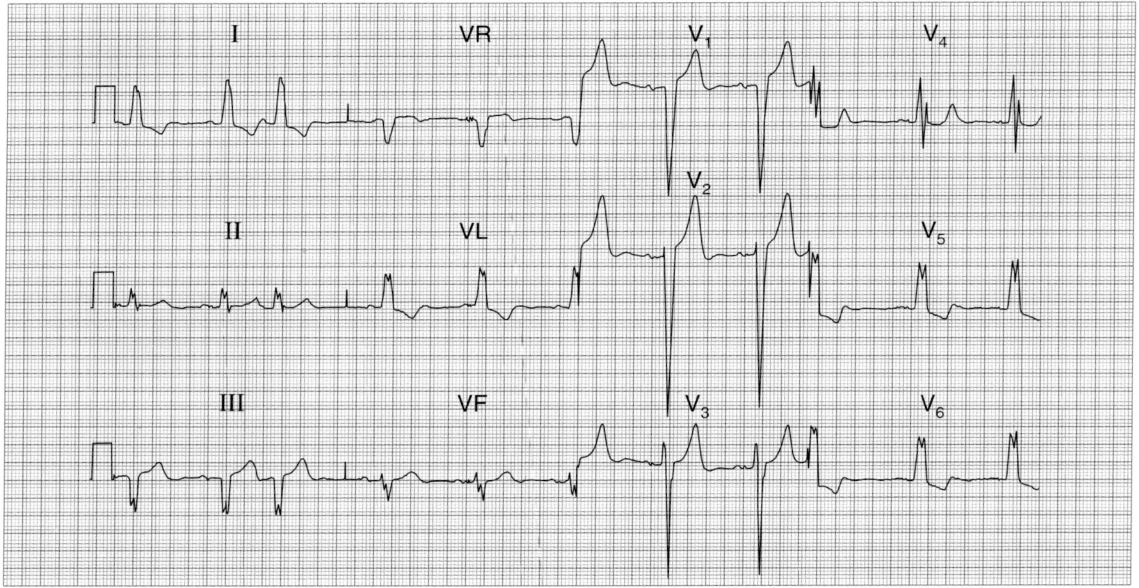

ECG 23 This ECG was recorded from a 70-year-old man who had had angina for some time and was treated with a beta-blocker. He came to the A & E department complaining of pain similar to his angina, but much more severe and persistent for 4 h. What does the ECG show and what treatment would be appropriate?

ANSWER 23

The ECG shows (*note*: leads at half sensitivity):

- Sinus rhythm
- Supraventricular (junctional) extrasystoles
- Normal axis
- Broad QRS complexes (140 ms)
- 'M' pattern of QRS complex in leads V_4–V_6
- Inverted T waves in leads I, VL, V_4–V_6

Clinical interpretation

This ECG shows sinus rhythm with supraventricular extrasystoles and left bundle branch block (LBBB). No further interpretation is possible.

What to do

If a patient has symptoms suggestive of a myocardial infarction of less than 6 h duration but has LBBB on the ECG, thrombolysis should be given only if the bundle branch block is known to be new. Here the patient had a history of angina so the first thing to do is to relieve his pain and the second is to find his old notes and see if the LBBB had been noted previously. If no old ECGs are available, thrombolysis should not be given, and the patient should be treated as an acute coronary syndrome. The supraventricular extrasystoles are not important.

Summary ★
Left bundle branch block; supraventricular extrasystoles.

ME See pp. 36 and 62

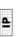

IP See p. 259

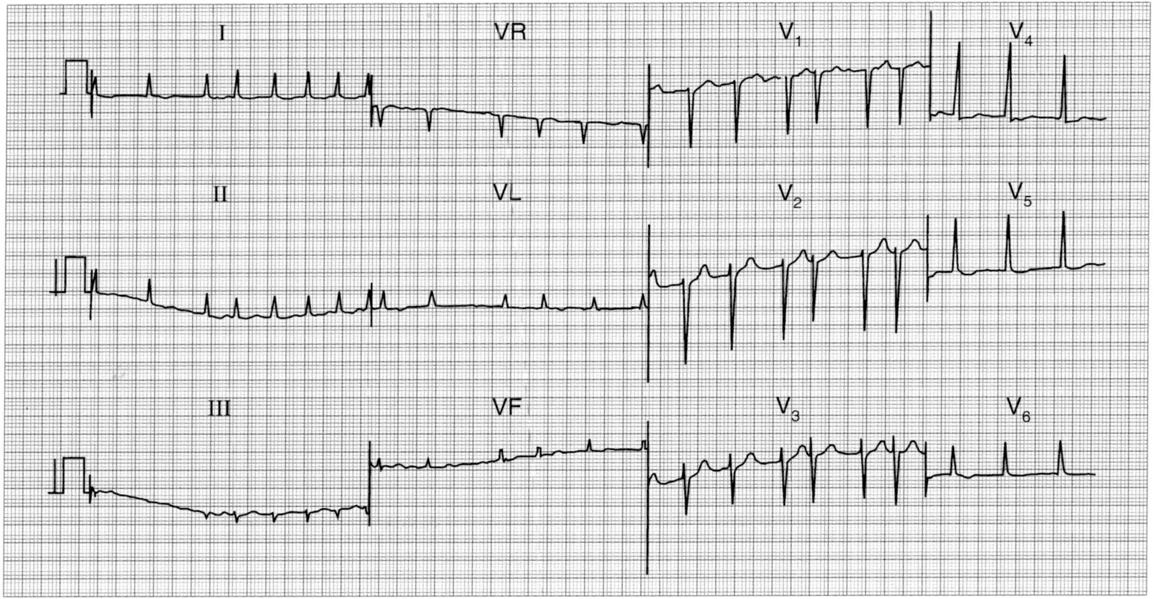

ECG 24 This ECG was recorded from a 60-year-old man being treated as an out-patient for severe congestive cardiac failure. What might be the diagnosis of the underlying heart condition and what would you do?

ANSWER 24

The ECG shows:

- Atrial fibrillation
- Ventricular rate 75–200/min
- Normal axis
- Normal QRS complexes
- Downward-sloping ST segment depression, especially in leads V_5, V_6

Clinical interpretation

The ventricular rate is not adequately controlled, though the ST segment depression suggests that he is taking digoxin. There are no changes to suggest ischaemia.

What to do

In the absence of clinical or ECG evidence of ischaemia, possible diagnoses include rheumatic heart disease, thyrotoxicosis, alcoholic heart disease, and other forms of cardiomyopathy. Echocardiography is necessary. The serum digoxin level must be checked and the digoxin dose increased if appropriate. In addition to digoxin, the patient will need an angiotensin-converting enzyme inhibitor, a diuretic and, probably, anticoagulants. Beta-blockers must be considered once his cardiac failure is controlled.

Summary ★★
Atrial fibrillation with an uncontrolled ventricular rate, and digoxin effect.

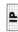

ME See pp. 78 and 107
IP See p. 315

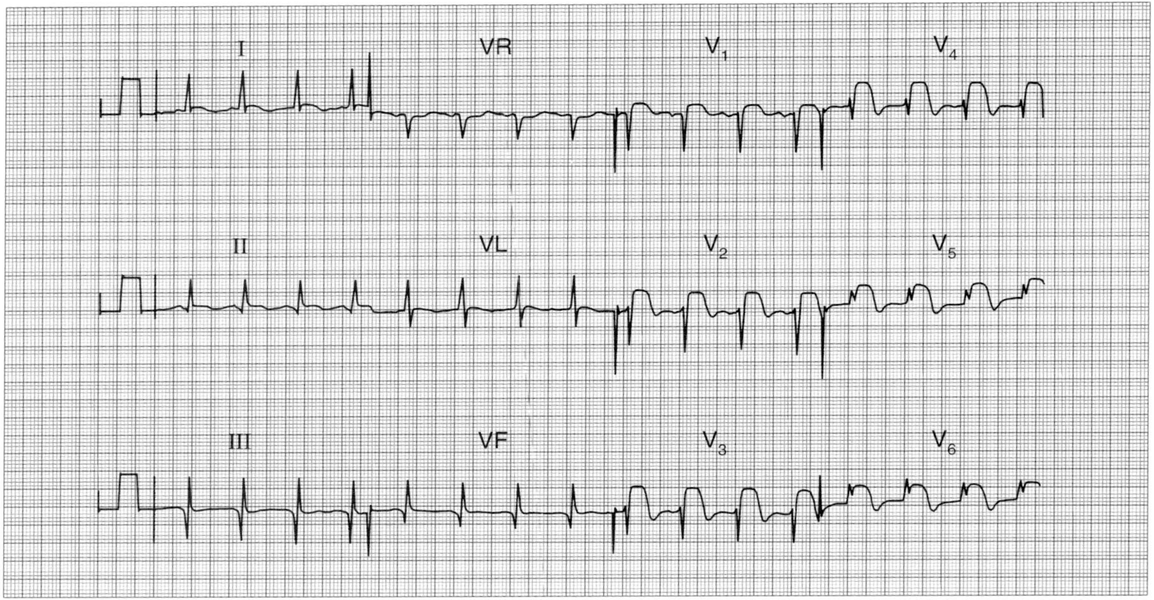

ECG 25 A 60-year-old man, who 3 years earlier had had a myocardial infarction followed by mild angina, was admitted to hospital with central chest pain that had been present for 1 h and had not responded to sublingual nitrates. What does his ECG show, and what would you do?

ANSWER 25

The ECG shows:

- Sinus rhythm
- Normal axis
- Q waves in leads II, III, VF
- Normal QRS complexes in the anterior leads
- Marked ST segment elevation in leads V_1–V_6

Clinical interpretation

The Q waves in leads III and VF suggest an old inferior infarction, while the elevated ST segments in leads V_1–V_6 indicate an acute anterior infarction.

What to do

The patient should be given pain relief, and in the absence of the usual contraindications should immediately be treated with aspirin and a thrombolytic agent. If he was treated with streptokinase for his previous infarction, he should be given alteplase or reteplase on this occasion.

Summary ★★

Old inferior and acute anterior myocardial infarctions.

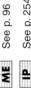

ME See p. 96

IP See p. 254

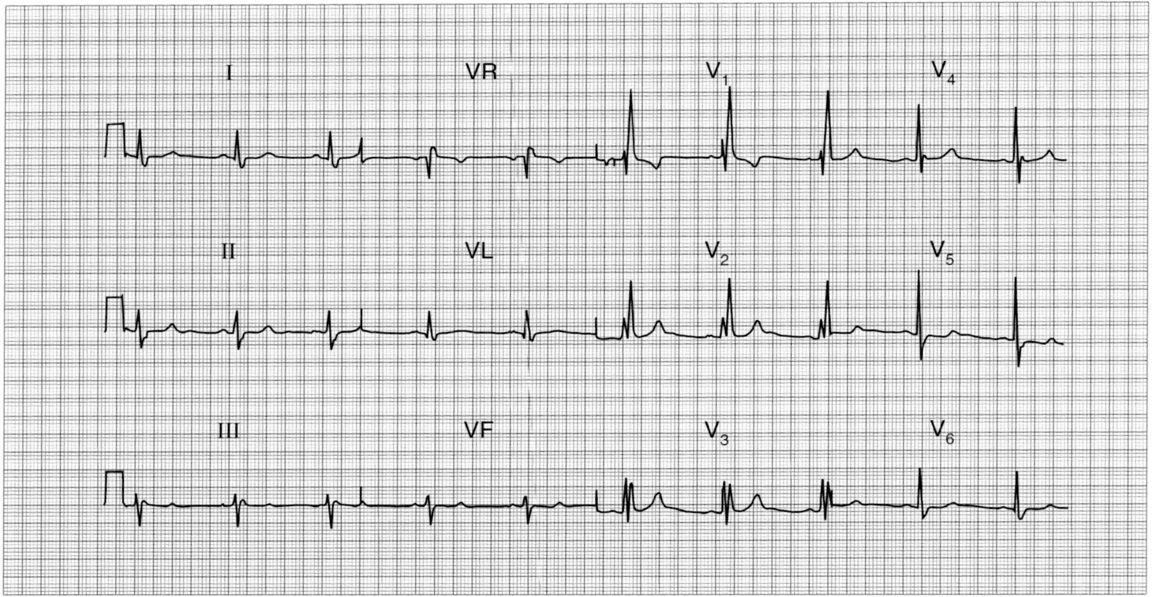

ECG 26 A 15-year-old boy was referred to the out-patient department because of a heart murmur. He had no symptoms. What does this ECG show and what physical signs would you look for?

ANSWER 26

The ECG shows:

- Sinus rhythm
- Normal axis
- Broad QRS complexes (140 ms)
- RSR pattern in lead I
- Wide and slurred S waves in lead V_5
- Normal ST segments and T waves

Clinical interpretation

Right bundle branch block.

What to do

Right bundle branch block is seen in a small proportion of people with perfectly normal hearts. In the presence of a heart murmur, however, the possibility of an atrial septal defect should be considered. This is what this patient had. The physical signs were a widely-split pulmonary second sound which did not vary with inspiration (this is typical of right bundle branch block) and an ejection systolic murmur best heard at the left sternal edge. On deep inspiration a soft diastolic murmur could be heard at the lower left sternal edge. The systolic murmur is a pulmonary flow murmur due to the extra flow through the right side of the heart, and the diastolic murmur that occurs on inspiration is a tricuspid flow murmur. The diagnosis was confirmed by echocardiography, and the defect was closed with a percutaneous 'umbrella' device. Following operation, the right bundle branch block persisted.

Summary ★
Sinus rhythm with right bundle branch block.

ME See p. 37

IP See pp. 103 and 352

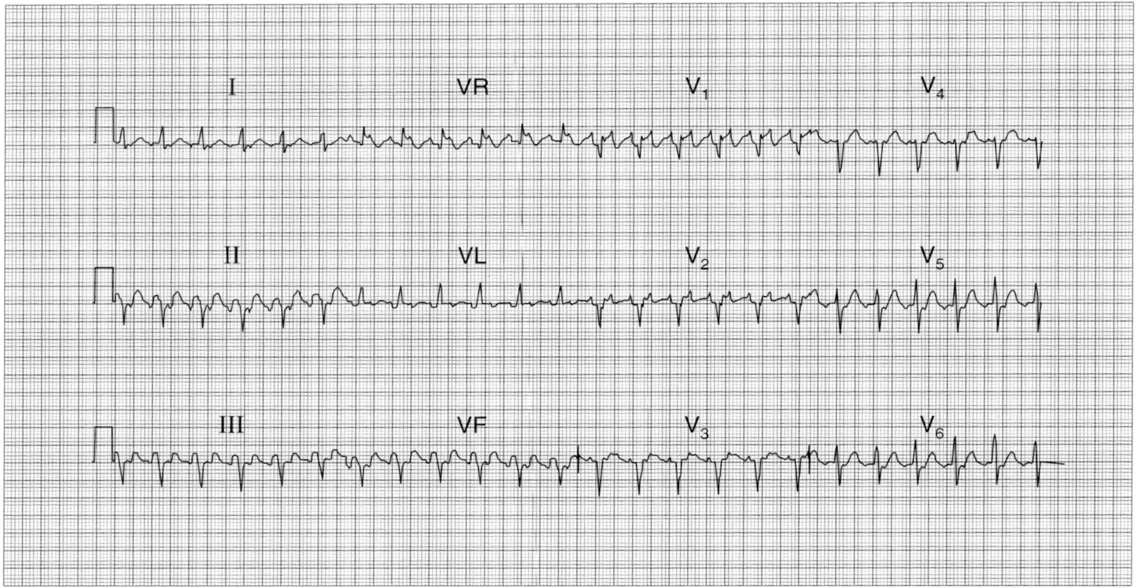

ECG 27 This ECG was recorded from a 40-year-old man who complained of breathlessness on climbing stairs. He was not aware of a fast heart rate and had had no chest pain. Apart from a rapid rate there were no cardiovascular abnormalities, but he looked a little jaundiced and had an enlarged spleen. What would you do?

ANSWER 27

The ECG shows:

- Atrial flutter
- Ventricular rate 140/min
- Left axis
- Normal QRS complexes, except that there is an S wave in lead V_6

Clinical interpretation

This ECG shows atrial flutter with 2:1 block. The left axis may be due to left anterior hemiblock, although the QRS has a normal duration so the significance of the axis is uncertain. The persistent S wave in lead V_6 suggests chronic lung disease.

What to do

Provided the patient is not in heart failure it is always a good idea to identify the cause of an arrhythmia before treating it. The combination of an atrial arrhythmia, jaundice and splenomegaly suggests alcoholism. The patient needs anticoagulants, but his international normalized ratio (INR) may already be high.

An echocardiogram is needed to assess left ventricular function, and digoxin could be given in an attempt to control the ventricular rate. After anticoagulation, cardioversion, either electrical or with flecainide, will be necessary.

Summary ★
Atrial flutter with 2:1 conduction.

ME See p. 68

IP See p. 160

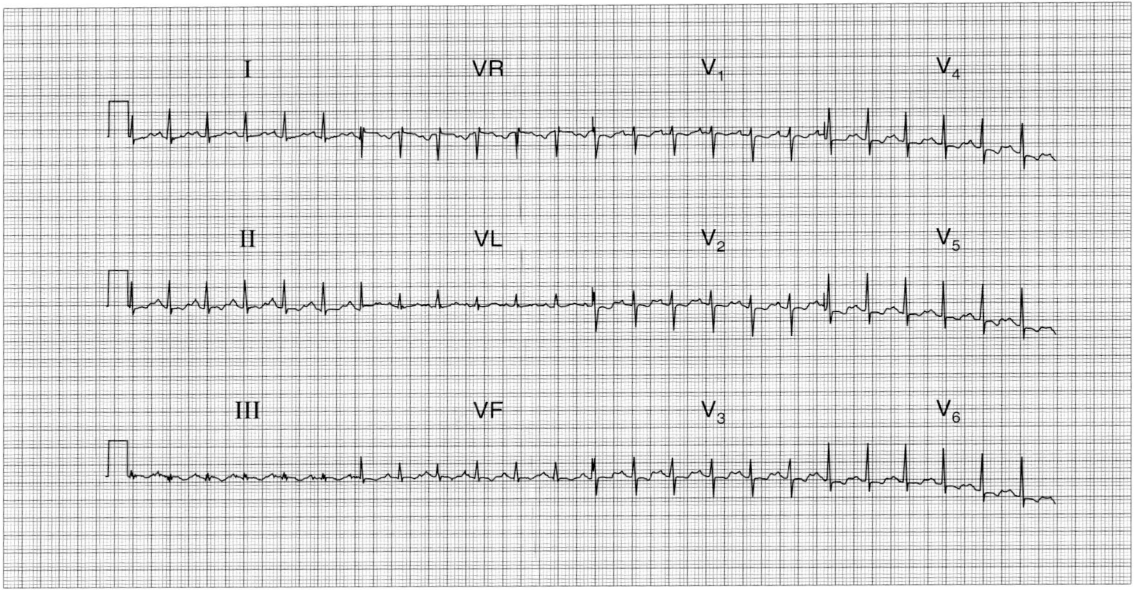

ECG 28 This ECG was recorded from a 39-year-old woman who complained of a sudden onset of breathlessness. She had no previous history, and no chest pain. Examination reveals nothing other than a rapid heart rate. What is the diagnosis?

ANSWER 28

The ECG shows:

- Sinus rhythm, rate 140/min
- Normal conduction
- Normal axis
- Normal QRS complexes
- Slightly depressed ST segments in leads V_1–V_4
- Biphasic or inverted T waves in the inferior and all the chest leads

Clinical interpretation

The ECG shows a marked sinus tachycardia, with no change in the cardiac axis and normal QRS complexes. The widespread ST/T changes are clearly very abnormal, but are not specific for any particular disease. However, the fact that leads V_1–V_3 are affected suggests a right ventricular problem.

What to do

This is a case where the ECG must be considered in the light of the patient's history and physical signs (if any). Clearly something has happened; the sudden onset of breathlessness without pain suggests a pulmonary embolus, and here the VQ scan confirmed multiple small pulmonary infarcts.

Summary ★★
Sinus tachycardia with widespread ST/T changes suggesting pulmonary embolism.

ME See p. 92
IP See p. 289

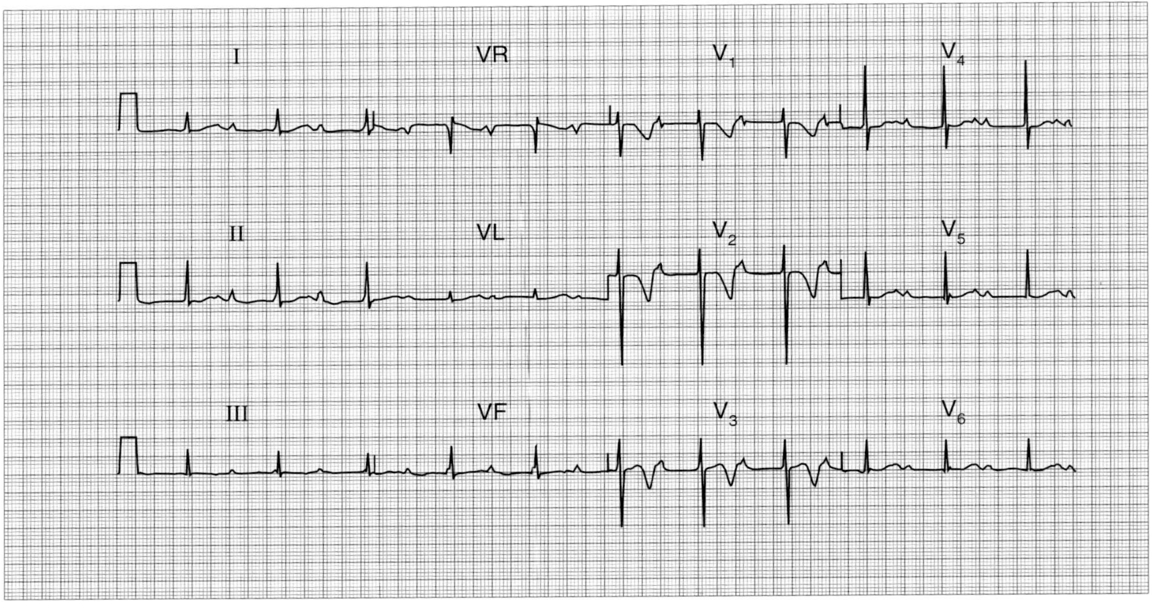

ECG 29 This ECG was recorded from a 50-year-old man who was admitted to hospital as an emergency, having had chest pain characteristic of a myocardial infarction for 3 h. What does the ECG show and how should the patient be treated?

ANSWER 29

The ECG shows:

- Sinus rhythm
- PR intervals markedly prolonged (480 ms)
- Normal axis
- Normal QRS complexes
- T wave inversion in leads V_1–V_3

Clinical interpretation

First degree block associated with a non-Q wave anterior myocardial infarction. Since the T wave inversion is in leads V_1–V_3 but not V_4 the possibility of a pulmonary embolus must be considered.

What to do

The changes on the ECG do not meet the conventional criteria for thrombolysis for myocardial infarction (raised ST segments or new left bundle branch block). First degree block is not an indication for temporary pacing, but the patient must be monitored in case higher degrees of block develop.

Summary ★★

First degree block and anterior non-Q-wave infarction.

ME See pp. 30 and 103

IP See p. 266

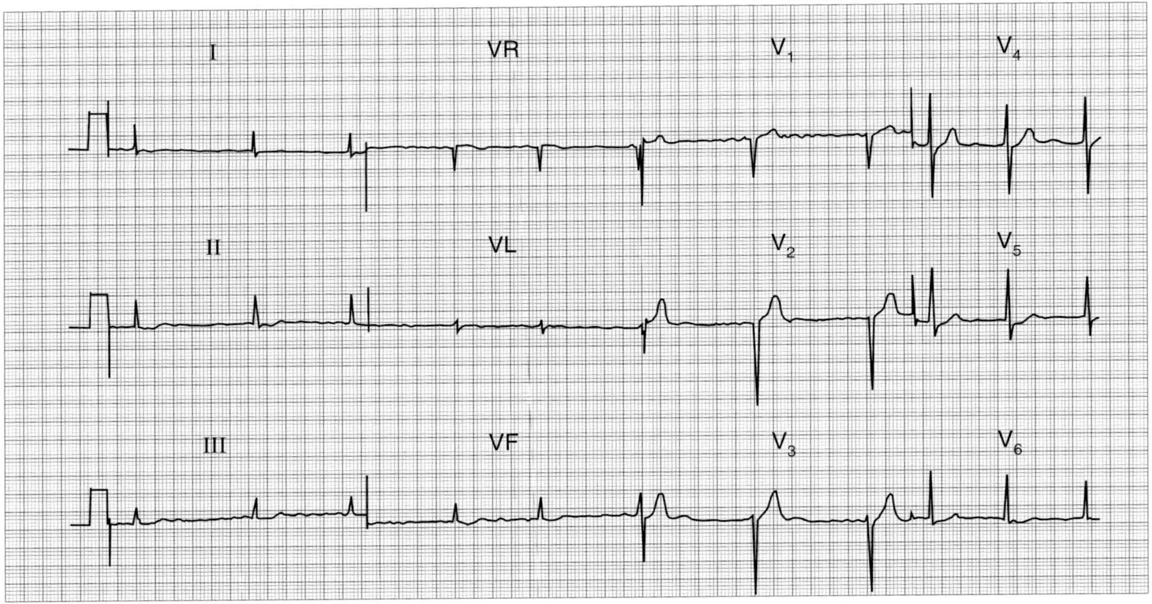

ECG 30 A 65-year-old man is seen in the out-patient department complaining of breathlessness and chest pain that has the characteristics of angina. He is untreated. Does his ECG help with his diagnosis and management?

ANSWER 30

The ECG shows:

- Atrial fibrillation
- Ventricular rate 50–70/min
- Normal axis
- Poor R wave progression (loss of R wave in lead V_3, with a normal R wave in lead V_4)
- Normal ST segments and T waves

Clinical interpretation

Normal ventricular rate, despite untreated atrial fibrillation. The poor R wave progression between leads V_3 and V_4 could result from inaccurate positioning of the chest leads, but may indicate an old anterior myocardial infarction.

What to do

Causes of atrial fibrillation other than ischaemia must be excluded. An exercise test will reveal whether or not his pain is angina, and will also show whether the ventricular rate remains controlled or whether it increases inappropriately.

Summary ★★

Atrial fibrillation and possible old anterior myocardial infarction.

ME See pp. 78 and 103

IP See pp. 243 and 251

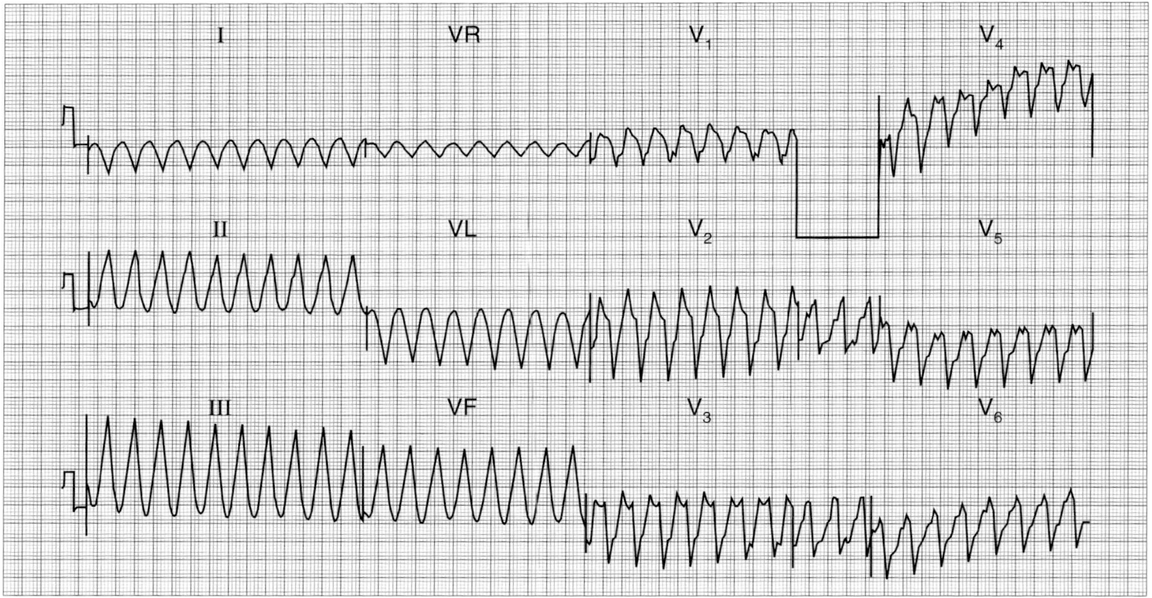

ECG 31 This ECG was recorded in a coronary care unit from a patient admitted 2 h previously with an acute anterior myocardial infarction. The patient was cold and clammy, and confused, and his blood pressure was unrecordable. What does the ECG show and what would you do?

ANSWER 31

The ECG shows:

- Broad-complex tachycardia, rate about 250/min
- Regular QRS complexes
- QRS duration 200 ms
- Indeterminate axis and QRS configurations

Clinical interpretation

In the context of acute myocardial infarction, broad-complex tachycardias should be considered to be ventricular in origin unless the patient is known to have bundle branch block when in sinus rhythm. Here the regularity of the rhythm and the very broad complexes of bizarre configuration leave no room for doubt that this is ventricular tachycardia.

What to do

In cases of severe circulatory failure, immediate DC cardioversion is needed.

Summary ★★★

Ventricular tachycardia.

ME See p. 72

IP See p. 178

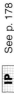

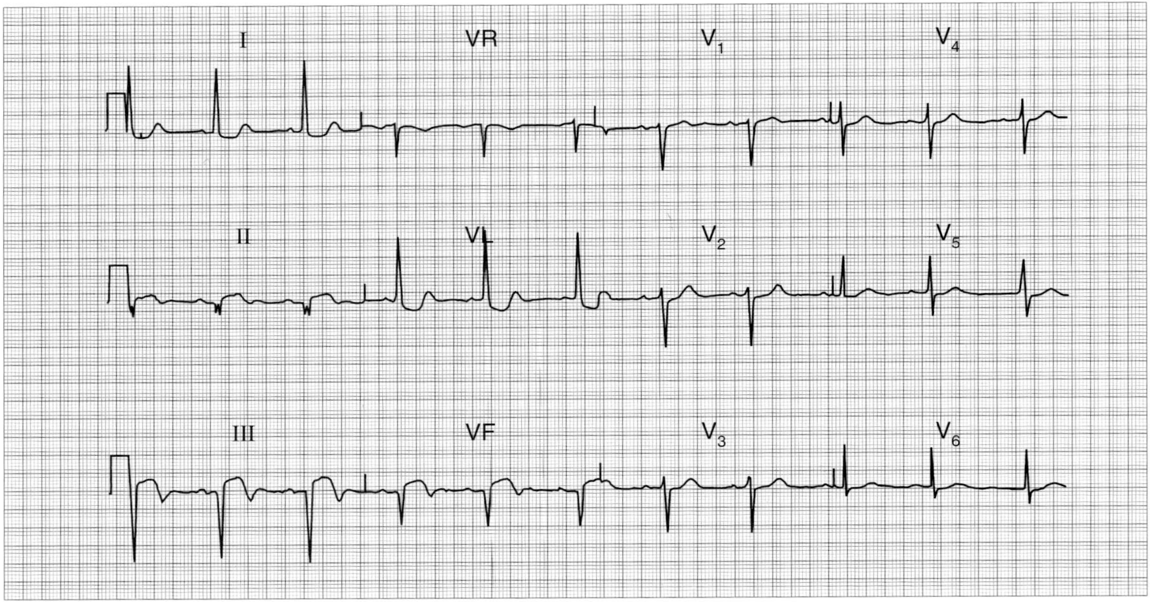

ECG 32 A 50-year-old man is admitted to hospital as an emergency, having had chest pain for 4 h. The pain is characteristic of a myocardial infarction. Apart from signs due to pain, the examination is normal. What does this ECG show and what would you do?

ANSWER 32

The ECG shows:

- Sinus rhythm
- Normal axis
- Q waves in leads II, III, VF
- Elevated ST segments in leads II, III, VF with biphasic T waves
- Downward-sloping ST segments in lead VL
- Normal QRS complexes, ST segments and T waves in the chest leads

Clinical interpretation

This is an acute inferior myocardial infarction. The rapidity of Q wave development is extremely variable, but the trace is certainly consistent with a 4 h history.

What to do

Pain relief is the most important part of the treatment. In the absence of contraindications, the patient should be given aspirin immediately, and then thrombolysis as soon as possible.

Summary ★
Acute inferior myocardial infarction.

ME See p. 96

IP See p. 242

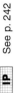

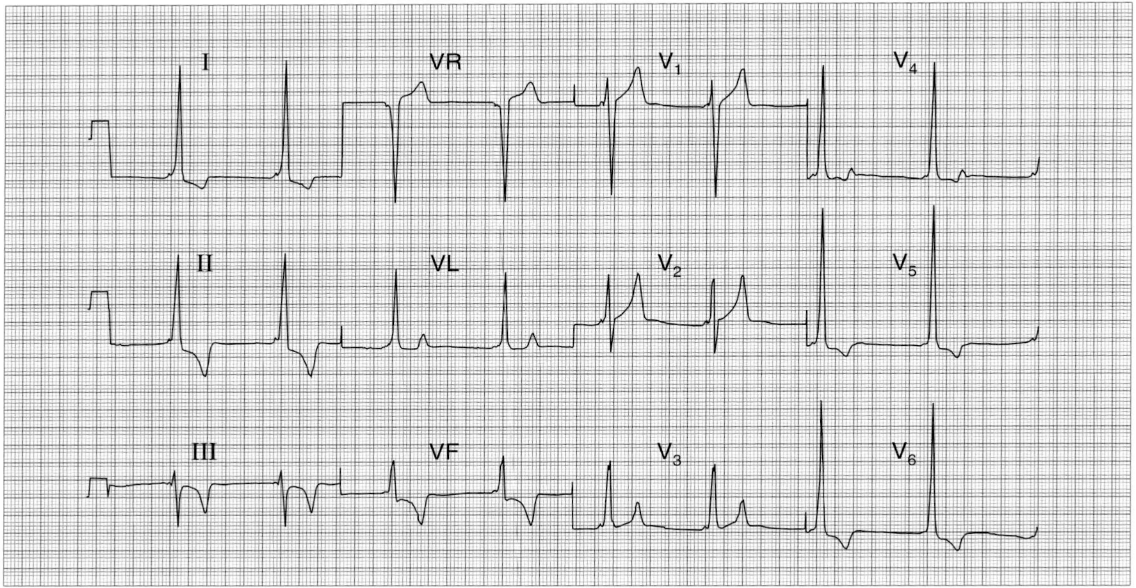

ECG 33 This ECG was recorded from a 35-year-old man who had no symptoms, but who had been found at a routine examination to have a blood pressure of 180/105. What does it show and what action would you suggest?

ANSWER 33

The ECG shows (*note*: leads at half sensitivity (0.5 cm = 1 mV)):

- Sinus rhythm, rate 50/min
- Very short PR interval
- Normal axis
- Slurred upstroke to QRS complexes – delta wave
- QRS duration prolonged (200 ms)
- Very tall QRS complexes in the lateral leads
- Inverted T waves in leads I, VL, III, VF, V_5–V_6

Clinical interpretation

This is an example of the Wolff–Parkinson–White syndrome type B. In a patient with high blood pressure the tall QRS complexes and inverted T waves in the lateral leads would raise the possibility of left ventricular hypertrophy, but the changes here are too gross for that, and they are compatible with this pre-excitation syndrome.

What to do

If the patient has no symptoms to suggest a paroxysmal tachycardia, no further action is necessary – many patients with pre-excitation on their ECG never have an episode of tachycardia.

Summary ★★

Wolff–Parkinson–White syndrome type B.

ME See p. 81

IP See pp. 38 and 104

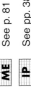

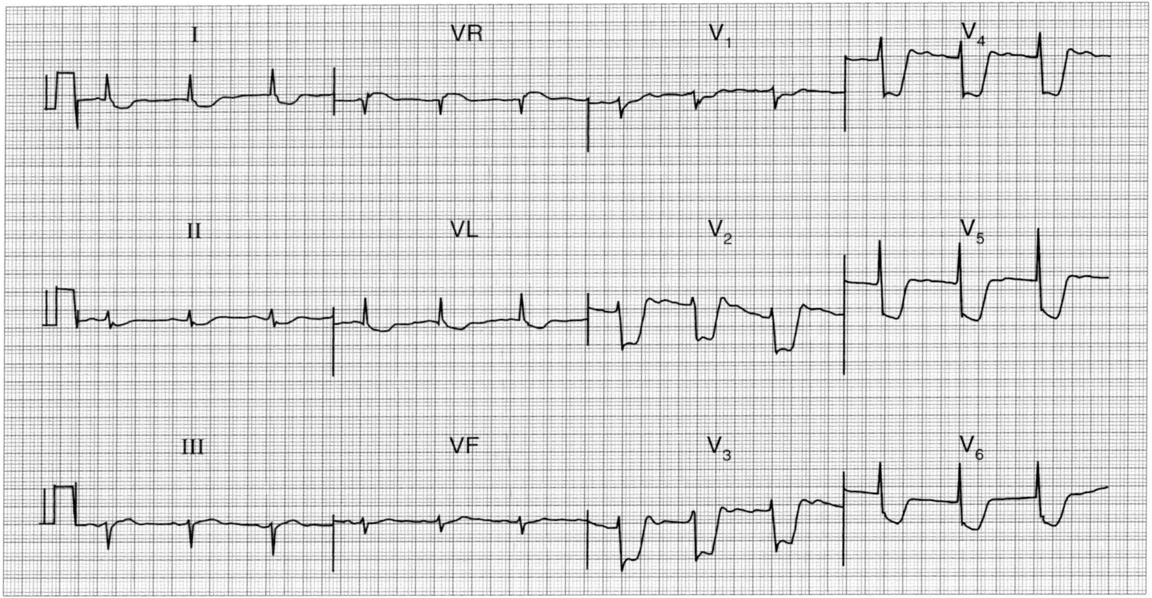

ECG 34 An 80-year-old man being observed in the recovery room following a femoral–popliteal bypass operation was noted to have an abnormal ECG. What does it show and what would you do?

ANSWER 34

The ECG shows:

- Sinus rhythm
- Normal axis
- Normal QRS complexes
- Marked (about 8 mm) horizontal ST segment depression in leads V_2–V_4, and downward-sloping ST segment depression in the lateral leads

Clinical interpretation

The patient is elderly and has peripheral vascular disease, so coronary disease is likely to be present. The appearance of the ECG is characteristic of severe cardiac ischaemia. The lack of a tachycardia is surprising.

What to do

This is not an easy situation to deal with because the patient's postoperative condition dictates management. He needs anticoagulation with aspirin and heparin, and intravenous nitrates should be given cautiously.

Summary ★★

Severe anterolateral ischaemia.

ME See p. 102

IP See p. 267

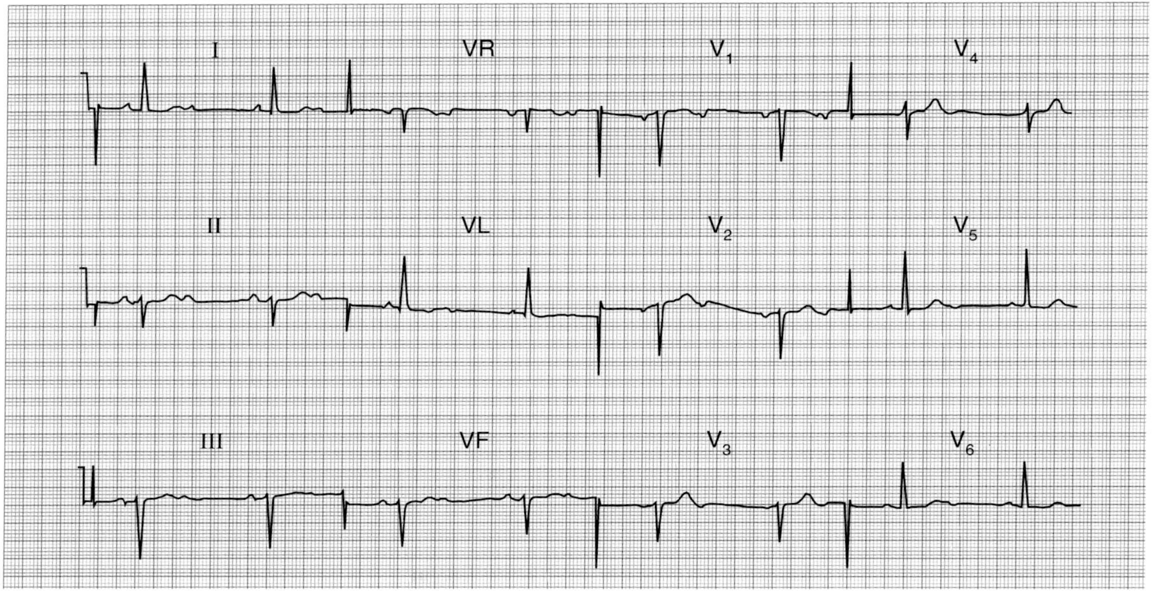

ECG 35 This ECG was recorded from a 75-year-old man who complained of breathlessness. He had not had any chest pain or dizziness. Apart from a slow pulse there were no abnormalities on examination. What three abnormalities are present in this record and how would you treat the patient?

ANSWER 35

The ECG shows:

- Sinus rhythm
- Second degree (2:1) block
- Left axis deviation
- Poor R wave progression in the anterior leads
- Normal T waves

Clinical interpretation

The second degree block is associated with a ventricular rate of 45/min, which may well be the cause of his breathlessness. The left axis deviation indicates left anterior hemiblock. The poor R wave progression (virtually no R wave in lead V_3, a small R wave in lead V_4, and a normal R wave in lead V_5) suggests an old anterior infarction.

What to do

This patient needs a permanent pacemaker.

Summary ★★★
Second degree (2:1) block, left anterior hemiblock, and probable old anterior infarction.

ME See pp. 31 and 46

IP See p. 140

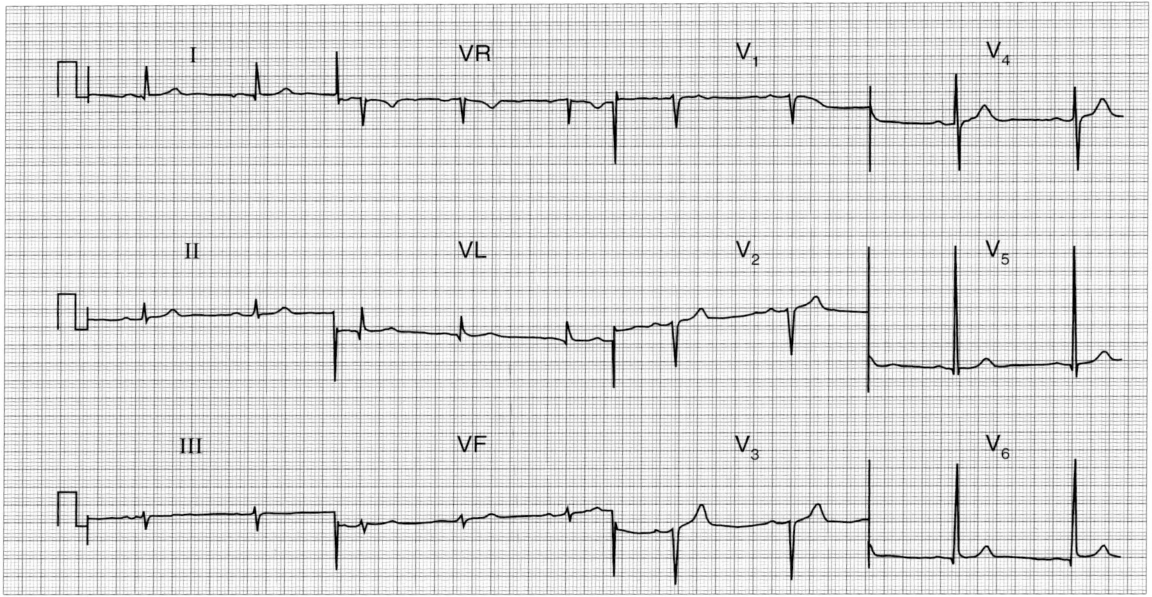

ECG 36 This ECG was recorded from a fit 22-year-old male medical student. He was worried – should he have been?

ANSWER 36

The ECG shows:

- Sinus rhythm
- Normal axis
- Tall R waves (28 mm in lead V_6, 32 mm in lead V_5)
- Loss of R waves in lead V_3
- Normal ST segments and T waves

Clinical interpretation

This record shows left ventricular hypertrophy by 'voltage criteria' (R waves greater than 25 mm in lead V_5 or V_6, or the sum of the R wave in lead V_5 or V_6 plus the S wave in lead V_1 or V_2 is greater than 35 mm). There are, however, no T wave changes. 'Voltage criteria' on their own are unreliable, and in a fit young man this may well be a normal variant. A loss of R waves in lead V_3 could indicate an old anterior infarction, but this is extremely unlikely in a young man and it probably results from faulty positioning of lead V_3.

What to do

Tell the student to buy a good book on ECG interpretation, but if reassurance is not enough, echocardiography could be used to measure left ventricular thickness.

Summary ★★

Left ventricular hypertrophy on 'voltage criteria', but probably normal.

ME See p. 93

IP See p. 68

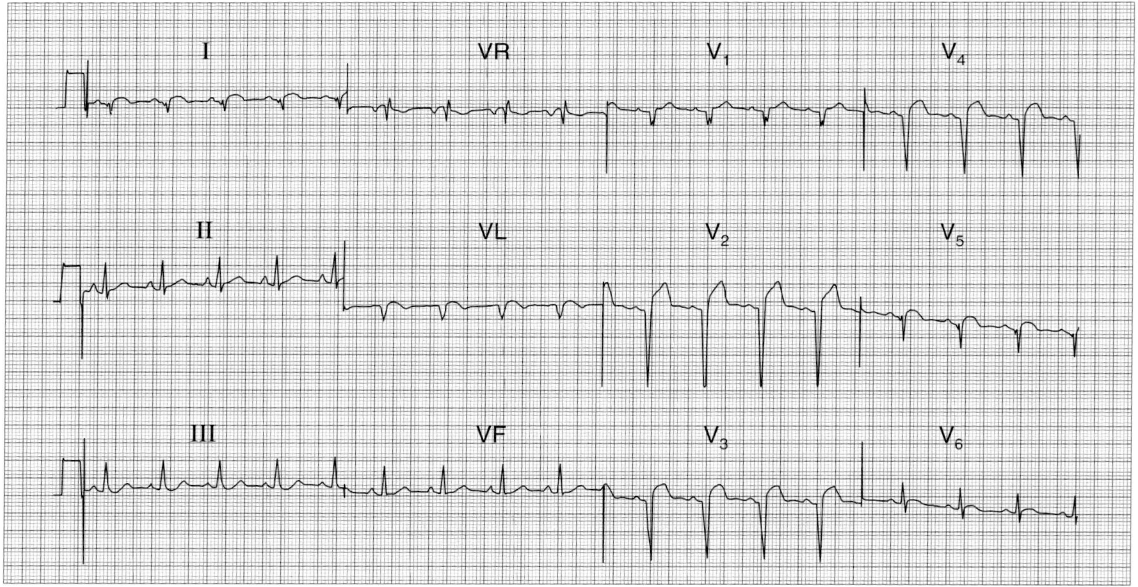

ECG 37 A 70-year-old man is seen as an out-patient with symptoms and signs of heart failure. His problem had begun quite suddenly a few weeks previously, when he had had a few hours of dull central chest discomfort. What does his ECG show and what would you do?

ANSWER 37

The ECG shows:

- Sinus rhythm, rate 100/min
- Normal axis
- Q waves in leads I, VL, V_2–V_5
- Raised ST segments in leads I, VL, V_2–V_6
- T wave inversion in lead V_6

Clinical interpretation

The raised ST segments suggest an acute infarction, but the deep Q waves suggest that the infarction occurred at least several hours previously. From the patient's story it seems clear that he had an infarction several weeks before he was seen, and there was nothing in the history to suggest a more recent episode. These ECG changes are therefore probably all old; the anterior changes might indicate a left ventricular aneurysm.

What to do

An ECG should always be interpreted in the light of the patient's clinical state. Since the ECG is compatible with an old infarction it should be assumed that this is the case, and the patient should be treated for heart failure in the usual way with diuretics, angiotensin-converting enzyme inhibitors and beta-blockers. Since the heart failure is clearly due to ischaemia he also needs aspirin and a statin.

Summary ★
Anterolateral myocardial infarction of uncertain age.

ME See p. 103
IP See p. 243

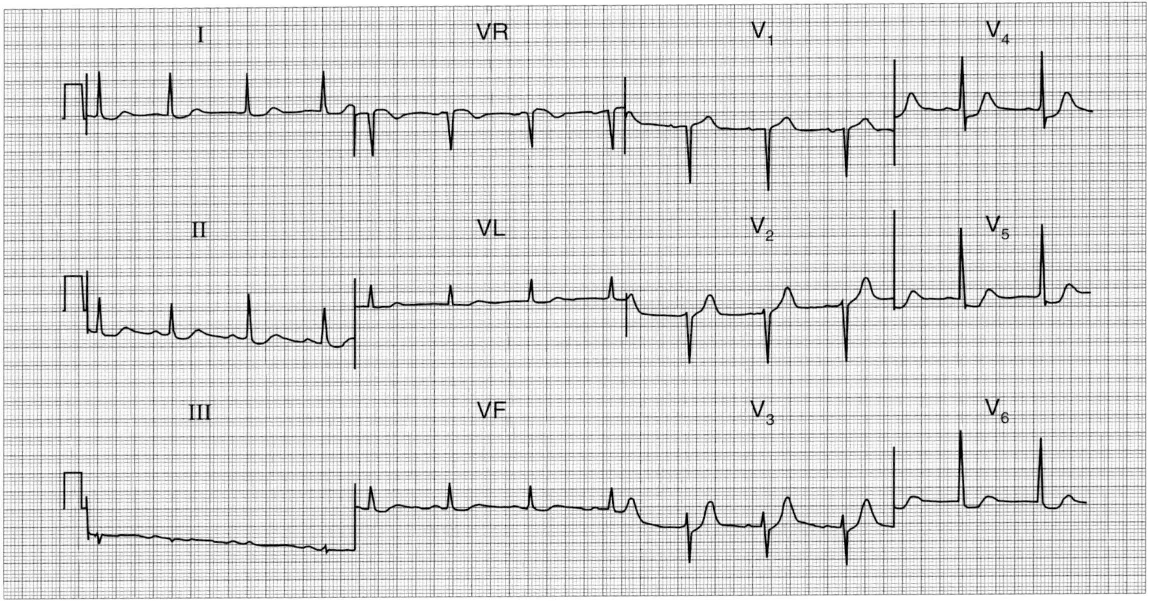

ECG 38 A 60-year-old man was referred to the out-patient department because of exercise-induced chest pain, and his GP had recorded this ECG. What does it show and what physical signs would you look for?

ANSWER 38

The ECG shows:

- Sinus rhythm
- Normal axis
- Normal QRS complexes
- Slight ST segment depression in leads I, II, VL
- 2–3 mm flat or downward-sloping ST segment depression in leads V_4–V_6

Clinical interpretation

The ST segment changes in leads I, II and VL are non-specific, but those in leads V_4–V_5 are undoubtedly due to ischaemia because the depression is horizontal and more than 2 mm. The downward-sloping ST segment in lead V_6 is also probably due to ischaemia, but could be due to digoxin.

What to do

There are no physical signs of angina, but there may be signs of pain (pallor, sinus tachycardia), heart failure (including a gallop rhythm at the cardiac apex), or there may be evidence of hypertension, hypercholesterolaemia, or smoking. There may be absent pulses or bruits over a peripheral artery, suggesting peripheral vascular disease. An exercise test would probably accentuate the ischaemic changes, but is not necessary for diagnostic purposes.

Summary ★★

ST segment depression due to ischaemia.

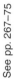

ME See p. 102

IP See pp. 267–75

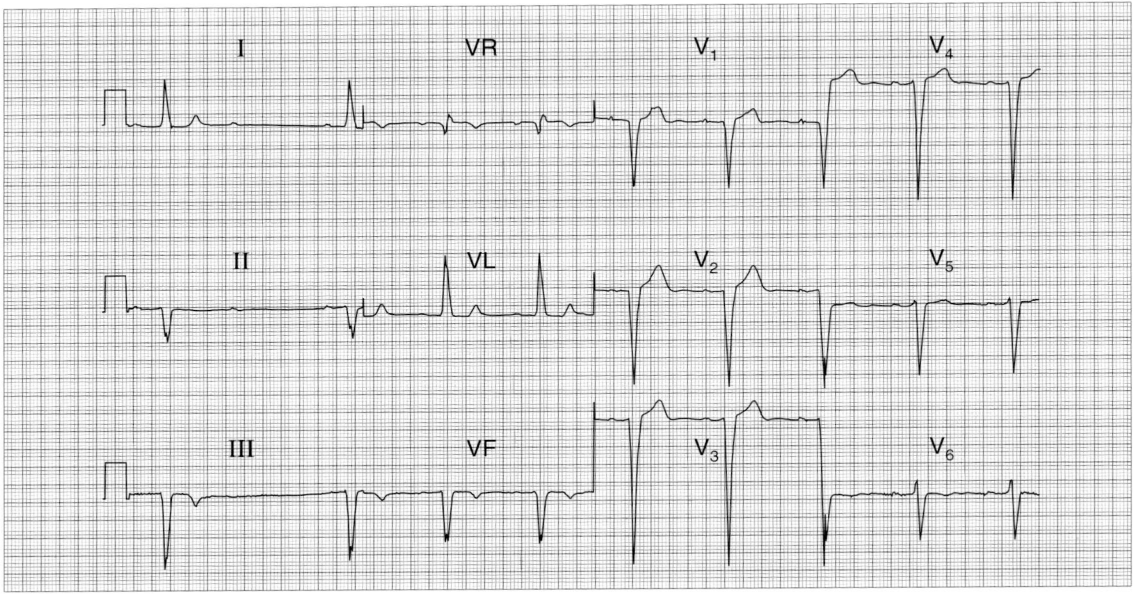

ECG 39 A 65-year-old man, who had had a myocardial infarction 3 years previously, presents with 2 h of chest pain that sounds ischaemic. By the time he was seen his pain had settled. What does his ECG show, what do you think has happened, and how should he be treated?

ANSWER 39

The ECG shows:

- Sinus rhythm
- Second degree block (Mobitz type 2 – best seen in leads I and II)
- Ventricular rate 50/min
- Normal PR interval in the conducted beats
- Left axis deviation
- Broad QRS complexes (160 ms)
- No R waves in anterior chest leads
- Deep S wave in lead V_6

Clinical interpretation

The combination of Mobitz type 2 block and left interior hemiblock (shown by the left axis) indicates severe conduction tissue disease. The loss of R waves in the chest leads may be due to an old anterior infarction, but the deep S wave in lead V_6 may indicate an intraventricular conduction delay.

What to do

The recent episode of chest pain may have been due to a further myocardial infarction, or may have been associated with bradycardia due to complete heart block. If repeat ECGs and blood markers suggest there has no infarction, then a permanent pacemaker is needed; if there is evidence of a new infarction it would be reasonable to monitor the patient closely and see if the heart block improves.

Summary ★★

Mobitz type 2 (second degree) block and left anterior hemiblock; probable old anterior infarction.

ME See pp. 31 and 46

IP See p. 140

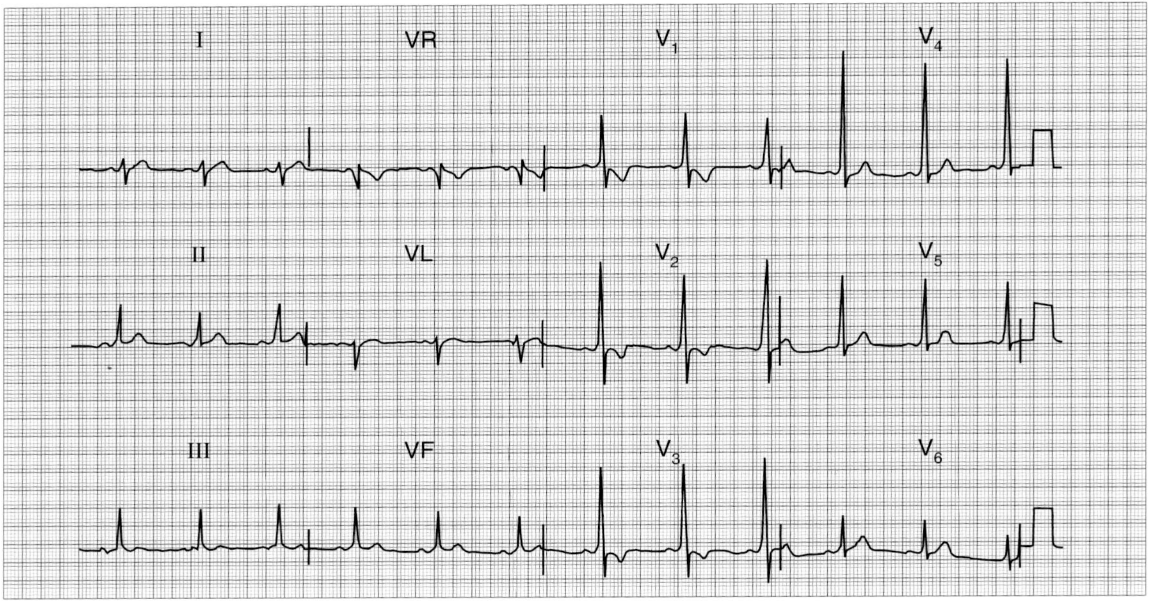

ECG 40 A 30-year-old woman, who had a normal pregnancy and delivery 3 months ago, complains of breathlessness but has no other symptoms. She has a soft systolic murmur, and this is her ECG. What does it show and what would you do?

ANSWER 40

The ECG shows:

- Sinus rhythm
- Normal axis
- Short PR interval, best seen in lead V_5
- Dominant R waves in lead V_1
- Slurred upstroke (delta wave) in the QRS complexes
- Inverted T waves in leads V_1–V_3

Clinical interpretation

This is the Wolff–Parkinson–White syndrome, involving a short PR interval and a widened QRS complex. This pattern, where there is a left-sided accessory pathway and which is called 'type A', can easily be mistaken for right ventricular hypertrophy.

What to do

The Wolff–Parkinson–White syndrome is unrelated to the pregnancy and delivery, and in the absence of symptoms suggesting an arrhythmia does not provide any explanation for breathlessness. No action is required as far as the Wolff–Parkinson–White syndrome is concerned, and other causes of breathlessness must be considered – for example, anaemia or pulmonary emboli.

Summary ★★
Wolff–Parkinson–White syndrome.

ME See p. 81
IP See p. 120

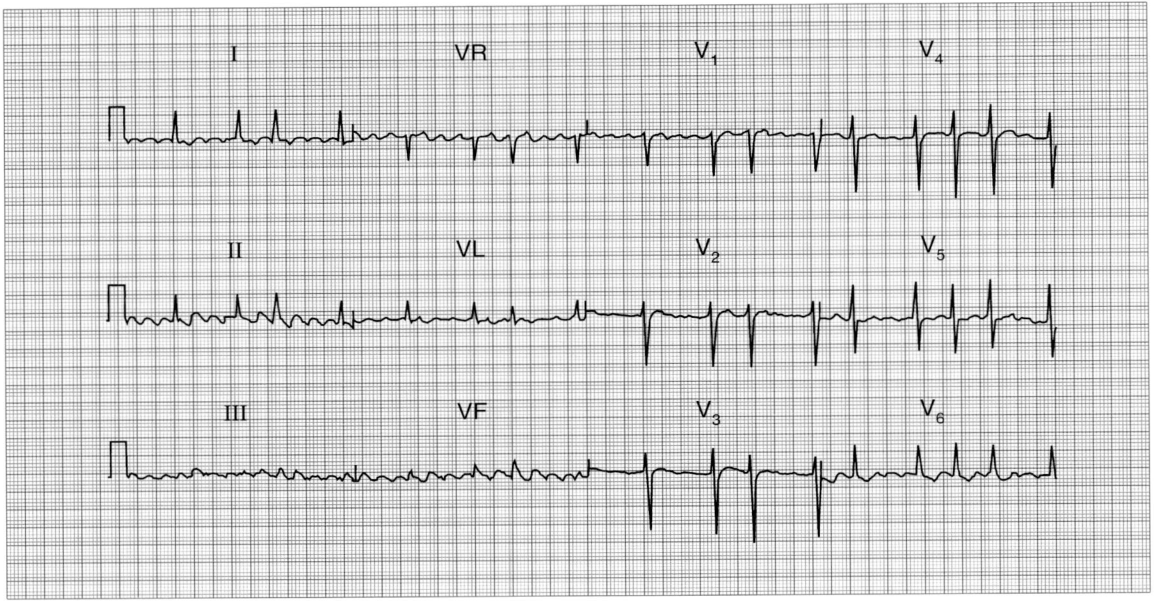

ECG 41 A 70-year-old woman, from whom this ECG was recorded, was admitted to hospital with increasing congestive cardiac failure. What does the ECG show and what would you do?

ANSWER 41

The ECG shows:

- Atrial fibrillation
- Normal axis
- Normal QRS complexes
- Downward-sloping ST segment depression in lead V_6

Clinical interpretation

The rhythm could be interpreted as atrial flutter, particularly in leads II and V_1. However, the flutter-like activity is variable, and the QRS complexes are completely irregular. The old-fashioned term for this was 'flutter fibrillation'. The ST segment depression suggests digoxin effect.

What to do

'Flutter fibrillation' has the characteristics of atrial fibrillation, and it is better simply to use this latter term. The ventricular rate in this case is fairly rapid, suggesting that the patient may not have been given adequate digoxin. It would be prudent to check her digoxin level before increasing the dose. The ventricular rate may well slow down after treatment for heart failure with an angiotensin-converting enzyme inhibitor and a diuretic. Some form of anticoagulation is necessary. The thyroid function tests should be checked.

Summary ★
Atrial fibrillation and digoxin effect.

ME See pp. 78 and 107

IP See p. 170

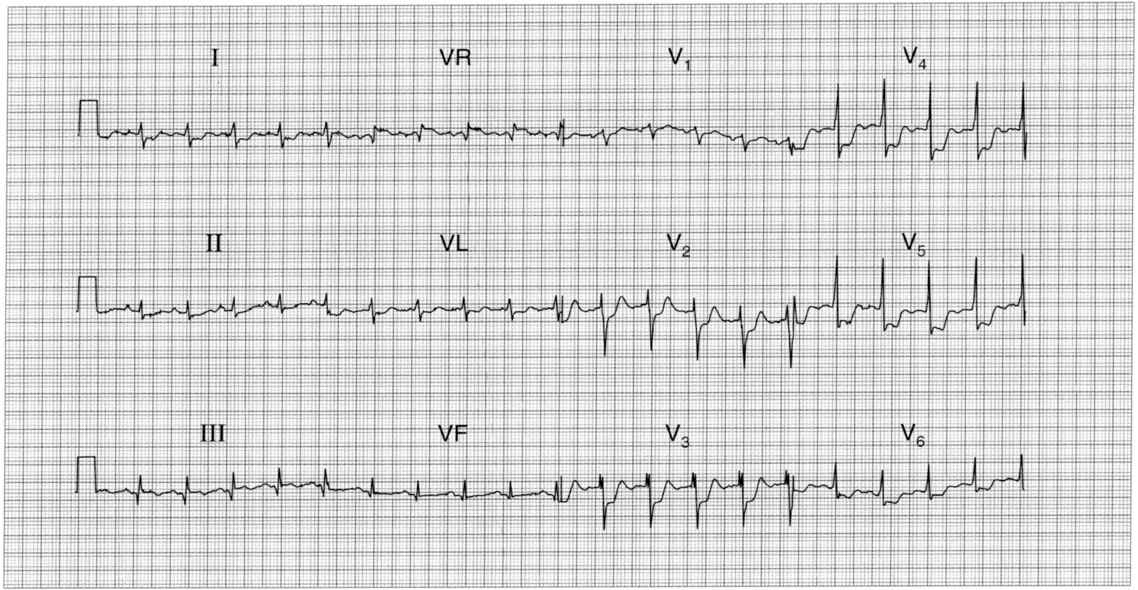

ECG 42 A 50 year old man, who had had exertional chest pain for some months, was seen in the A & E department with an hour of persistent central chest pain, and this is his ECG. What does the ECG show and what would you do?

ANSWER 42

The ECG shows:

- Sinus rhythm, rate 120/min
- Normal axis
- Small Q waves in leads III, VF
- 'Splintered' QRS complex in lead V_3; normal QRS complex duration (100 ms)
- Marked ST segment depression, horizontal in leads V_3, V_4 and downward-sloping in leads V_5, V_6
- ST segment depression is 5 mm in lead V_3
- T waves normal

Clinical interpretation

The sinus tachycardia is consistent with the patient's pain. The horizontal or downward-sloping ST segment depression indicates anterior ischaemia. The small Q waves in the inferior leads, and the 'splintered' QRS complex in the anterior leads, are probably of no significance.

What to do

This patient clearly has an acute coronary syndrome ('unstable angina'). Thrombolysis is not indicated with ST segment depression. He needs a beta-blocker and a nitrate (intravenous or buccal), and may need diamorphine. The ECG should be recorded every half hour to see if ST segment elevation appears. He may well need early coronary angiography with a view to coronary intervention (percutaneous transluminal coronary angioplasty (PTCA) or coronary artery bypass graft (CABG)).

Summary ★
Anterior ischaemia.

ME See p. 102
IP See p. 267

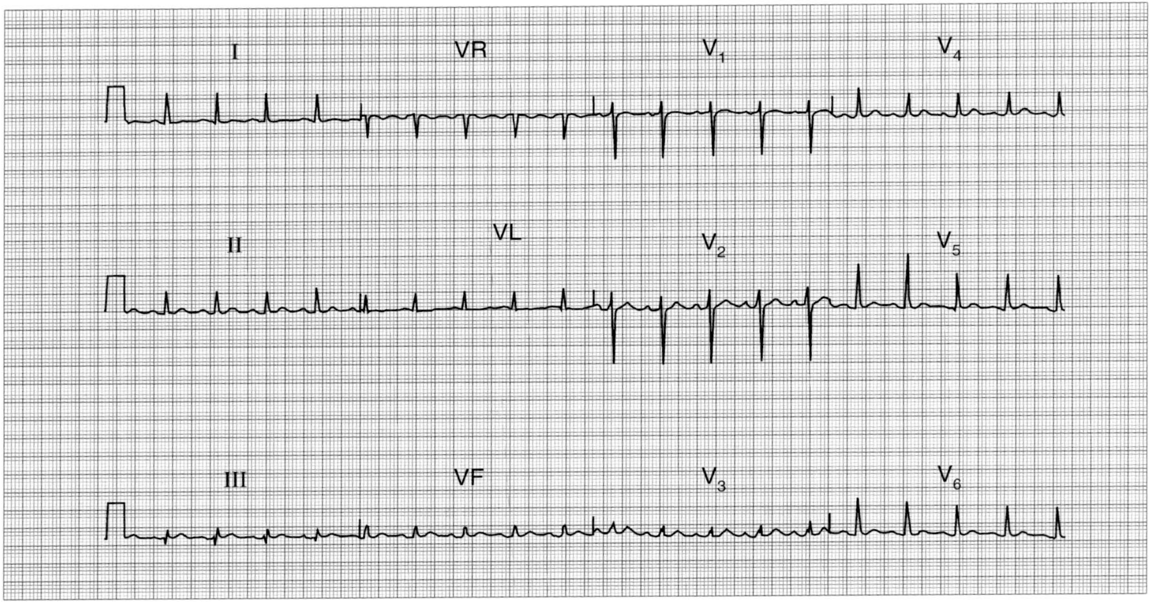

ECG 43 This ECG was recorded from a 30-year-old woman who complained of palpitations. Does it help make a diagnosis?

ANSWER 43

The ECG shows:

- Sinus rhythm, rate 110/min
- Normal axis
- Small Q waves in lead III
- Otherwise, normal QRS complexes and T waves

Clinical interpretation

Small Q waves in lead III but not in lead VF are normal. In establishing the cause of palpitations the history and examination are vital, and the ECG is not often helpful unless it is recorded when the patient has symptoms. A persistent sinus tachycardia, as shown here, may be due to anxiety, thyrotoxicosis, acute blood loss, anaemia, or heart failure. This patient had thyrotoxicosis.

What to do

Treat the underlying cause of the sinus tachycardia.

Summary ★★
Sinus tachycardia.

ME See p. 54

IP See p. 152

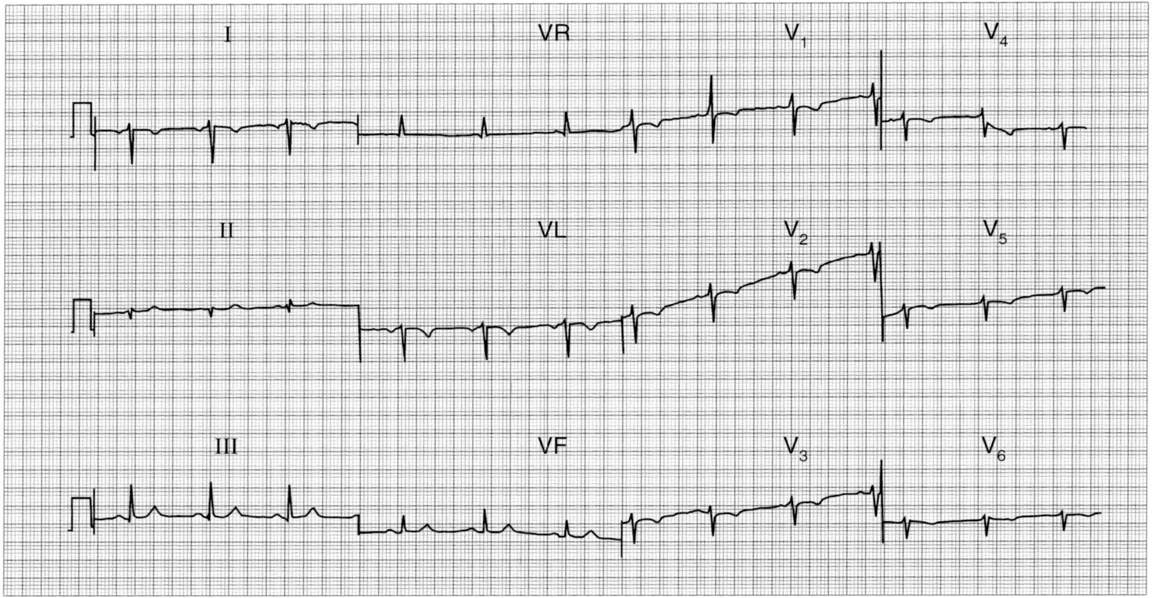

ECG 44 This ECG was recorded from a healthy 25-year-old man during a routine medical examination. Any comments?

ANSWER 44

The ECG shows:

- A very odd appearance
- Sinus rhythm
- Inverted P waves in lead I
- Right axis deviation
- Normal width QRS complexes
- Dominant R waves in lead VR
- No R wave development in the chest leads, with lead V_6 still showing a right ventricular pattern

Clinical interpretation
This is dextrocardia. A normal trace would be obtained with the limb leads reversed and the chest leads attached in the usual rib spaces but on the right side of the chest.

What to do
Ensure that the leads were properly attached – for example inverted P waves in lead I will be seen if the right and left arm attachments are reversed. Of course this would not affect the appearance of the ECG in the chest leads.

Summary ★★★
Dextrocardia.

IP See pp. 57 and 60

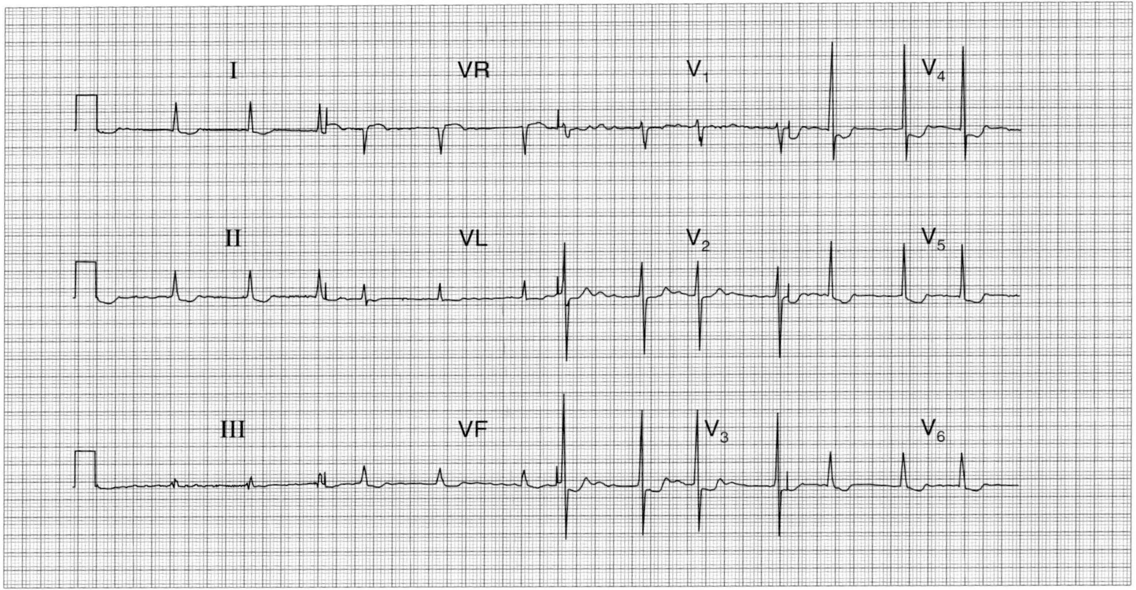

ECG 45 An 80-year-old woman, who has apparently been treated for heart failure for years, complains of nausea and vomiting. No previous records are available. Does her ECG help her management?

ANSWER 45

The ECG shows:

- Atrial fibrillation, ventricular rate 80/min
- Normal axis
- Normal QRS complexes
- Downward-sloping ST segment depression, especially in leads V_4–V_6
- T waves probably upright

Clinical interpretation

The ECG shows atrial fibrillation with a controlled ventricular rate. There is nothing on the ECG to suggest a cause for the arrhythmia or the patient's heart failure. The 'reversed tick' ST segment depression suggests that she is being treated with digoxin. The ECG does not suggest digoxin toxicity, but nevertheless this is the most likely cause for her nausea.

What to do

Digoxin therapy should be temporarily discontinued, and her plasma potassium and digoxin levels should be checked.

Summary ★

Atrial fibrillation and the digoxin effect.

ME See pp. 78 and 107

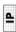

IP See p. 372

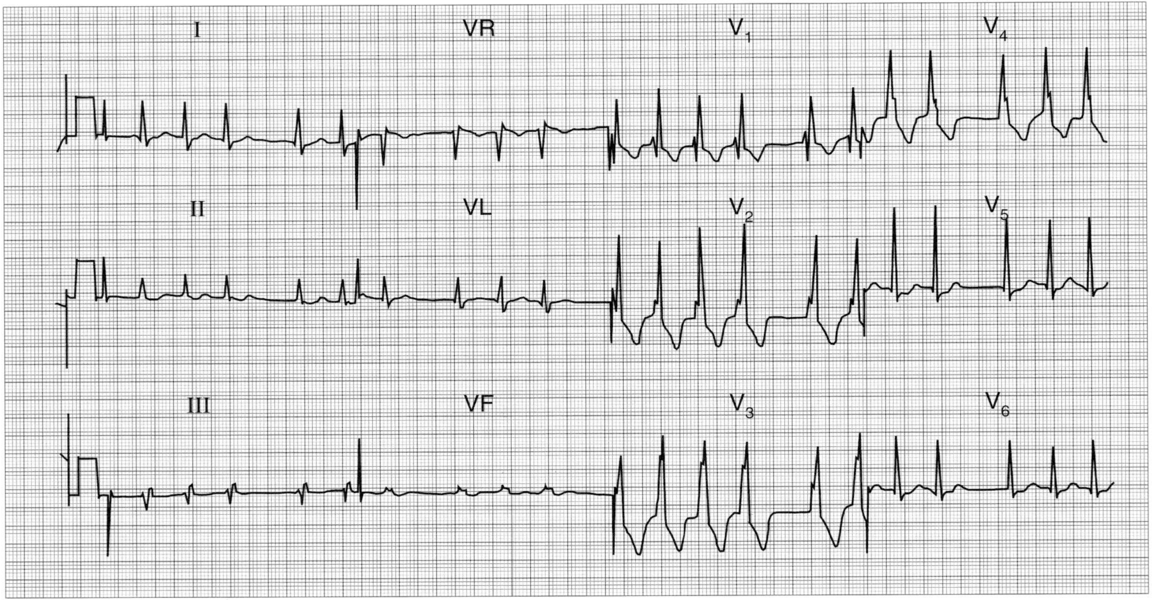

ECG 46 A 60-year-old man, whose heart and preoperative ECG had been normal, developed a cough with pleuritic chest pain a few days after a cholecystectomy. This is his ECG: what does it show and what would you do?

ANSWER 46

The ECG shows:

- Atrial fibrillation
- Normal axis
- Right bundle branch block

Clinical interpretation

In this ECG the usual 'irregular baseline' of atrial fibrillation is not apparent, but the QRS complexes are so irregular that this must be the rhythm. The rhythm change, together with the development of right bundle branch block, could be due to a chest infection but is more likely to have been caused by a pulmonary embolus.

What to do

In a postoperative patient, anticoagulation can always cause haemorrhage. Nevertheless, the risk of death from a pulmonary embolus is so high that the patient should immediately be given heparin while steps are taken (chest X-ray examination, white blood cell count, sputum culture, lung scan) to differentiate between a chest infection and a pulmonary embolus.

Summary ★★★
Atrial fibrillation with right bundle branch block.

ME See pp. 36 and 78

IP See p. 289

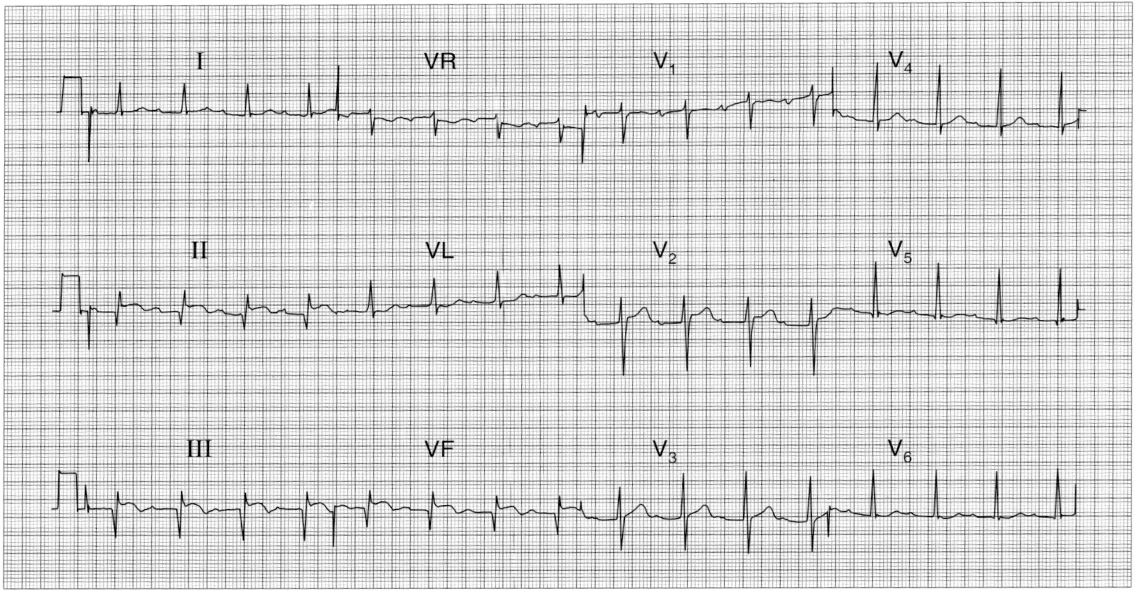

ECG 47 This ECG was recorded in the A & E department from a 50-year-old man with severe central chest pain that radiated into his back. The pain had been present for 6 h. What does the ECG show and what would you do?

ANSWER 47

The ECG shows:

- Sinus rhythm
- PR interval 320 ms – first degree block
- Q waves in leads II, III, VF
- Raised ST segments in leads II, III, VF
- Inverted T waves in leads III, VF

Clinical interpretation
This ECG shows an acute inferior myocardial infarction, which often causes first degree block. The Q waves and raised ST segments are consistent with the story of 6 h of chest pain, and the first degree block is not important.

What to do
Chest pain radiating through to the back has to raise the possibility of aortic dissection, which can occlude the opening of the coronary arteries and so cause a myocardial infarction. However, this is relatively rare whereas back pain associated with myocardial infarction is common. If nothing in the history or physical examination suggests a dissection, a thrombolytic should be given.

Summary ★
Acute myocardial infarction with first degree block.

ME See pp. 30 and 100

IP See p. 242

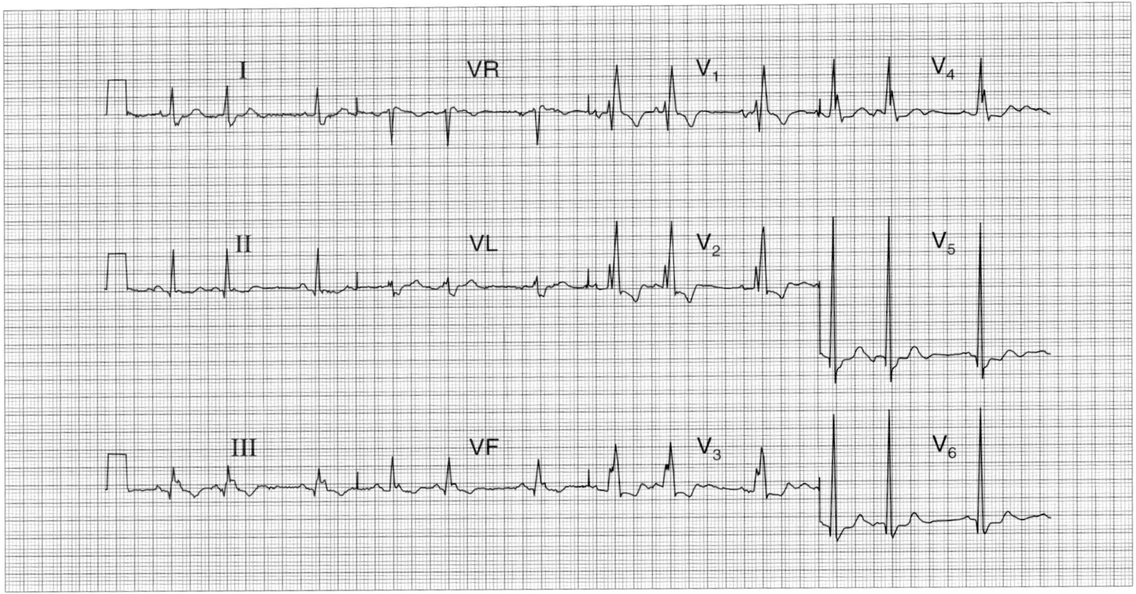

ECG 48 This ECG was recorded from a 23-year-old pregnant woman who had been found to have a heart murmur. What does it show and what might be the problem?

ANSWER 48

The ECG shows:

- Sinus rhythm
- Supraventricular (atrial) extrasystoles
- Normal PR interval
- Normal axis
- Wide QRS complex (160 ms)
- RSR pattern in lead V_1
- Broad slurred S wave in lead V_6
- Inverted T waves in leads V_1–V_3

Clinical interpretation

The broad QRS complex with an RSR pattern in lead V_1 and a slurred S wave in lead V_6, together with the inverted T waves in leads V_1–V_3 indicate right bundle branch block. The extrasystoles are supraventricular because they have the same (abnormal) QRS pattern as the sinus beats; they are atrial in origin because each is preceded by a T wave of slightly different shape from the sinus beats.

What to do

The palpitations of which the patient complains may well be due to the extrasystoles: it is important to ensure that they correspond to her symptoms. Right bundle branch block in a young person may indicate an atrial septal defect, and she should have an echocardiogram. The heart murmur could be due to a septal defect, but could well be a 'flow murmur' due to the increased cardiac output associated with pregnancy.

Summary ★
Right bundle branch block and atrial extrasystoles.

ME See pp. 36 and 62

IP See pp. 351–2

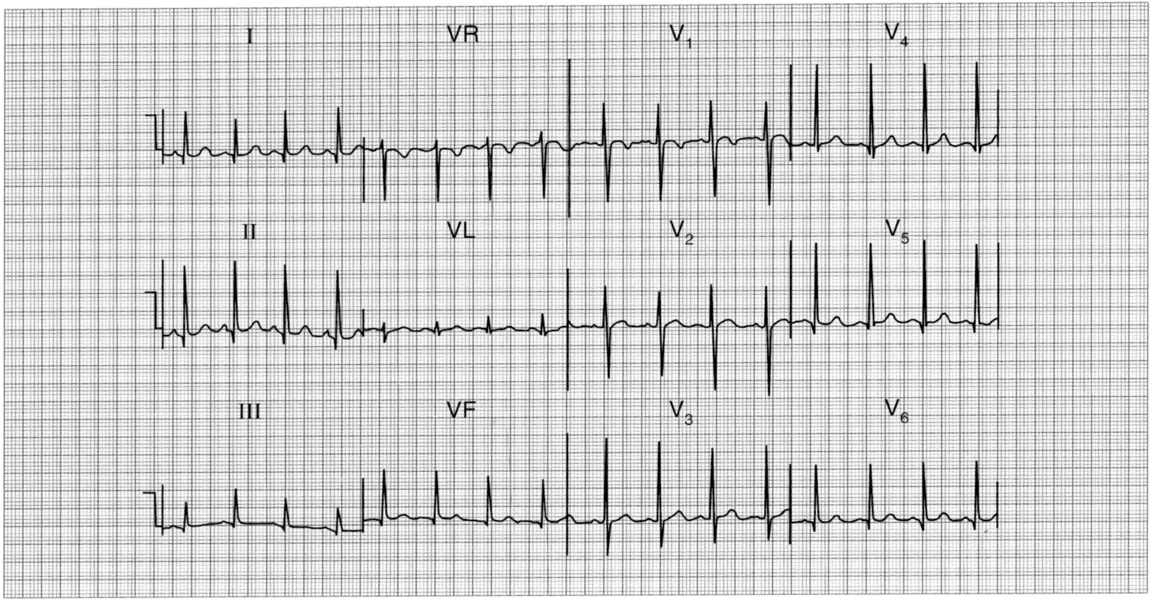

ECG 49 This ECG was recorded from a 9-year-old girl who was asymptomatic but who had been found to have a heart murmur at a school medical examination. What does it tell you about the murmur?

ANSWER 49

The ECG shows:

- Sinus rhythm, rate 100/min
- Normal axis
- Normal QRS complexes, but narrow, deep Q waves in leads I, II, V_4–V_6
- Inverted T waves in lead V_1

Clinical interpretation

A sinus tachycardia with normal QRS complexes, showing prominent 'septal' Q waves, is characteristic of ECGs of children. The inverted T wave in lead V_1 is normal at any age. A normal ECG helps to exclude serious causes of heart murmurs, but the record has not been very helpful in this case.

What to do

If in doubt, an echocardiogram will show whether there is any important structural abnormality in the heart.

Summary ★★

Normal ECG in a 9-year-old child.

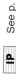

IP See p. 102

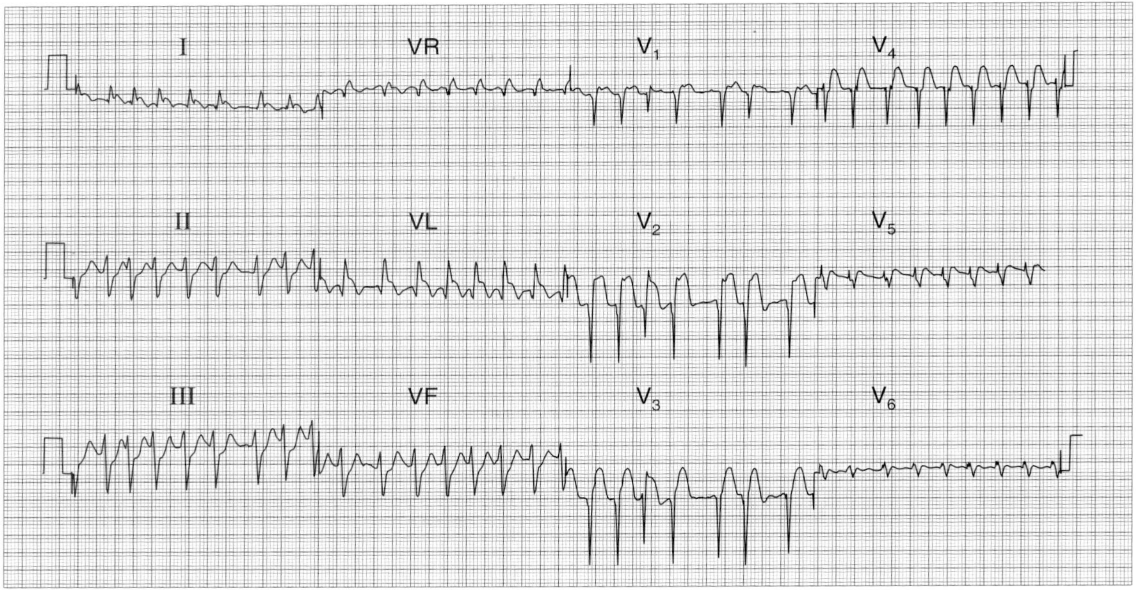

ECG 50 This ECG was recorded from a diabetic man who was admitted because of the sudden onset of pulmonary oedema. What do you think has happened?

ANSWER 50

The ECG shows:

- Atrial fibrillation with a ventricular rate of about 180/min
- Left axis
- QRS complexes of normal width and height
- Probable Q waves in leads V_2–V_4
- Raised ST segments in leads I, VL, V_2–V_4

Clinical interpretation

This ECG shows uncontrolled atrial fibrillation with left anterior hemiblock and an acute anterolateral myocardial infarction. The onset of atrial fibrillation may have been the cause or the consequence of the myocardial infarction, and the rapid ventricular rate will at least in part explain the pulmonary oedema. The left anterior hemiblock is probably a consequence of the infarction. The patient may not have experienced pain because of his diabetes.

Summary ★★

Atrial fibrillation, left anterior hemiblock and acute anterolateral myocardial infarction.

ME See pp. 46, 78 and 98

IP See pp. 246 and 315

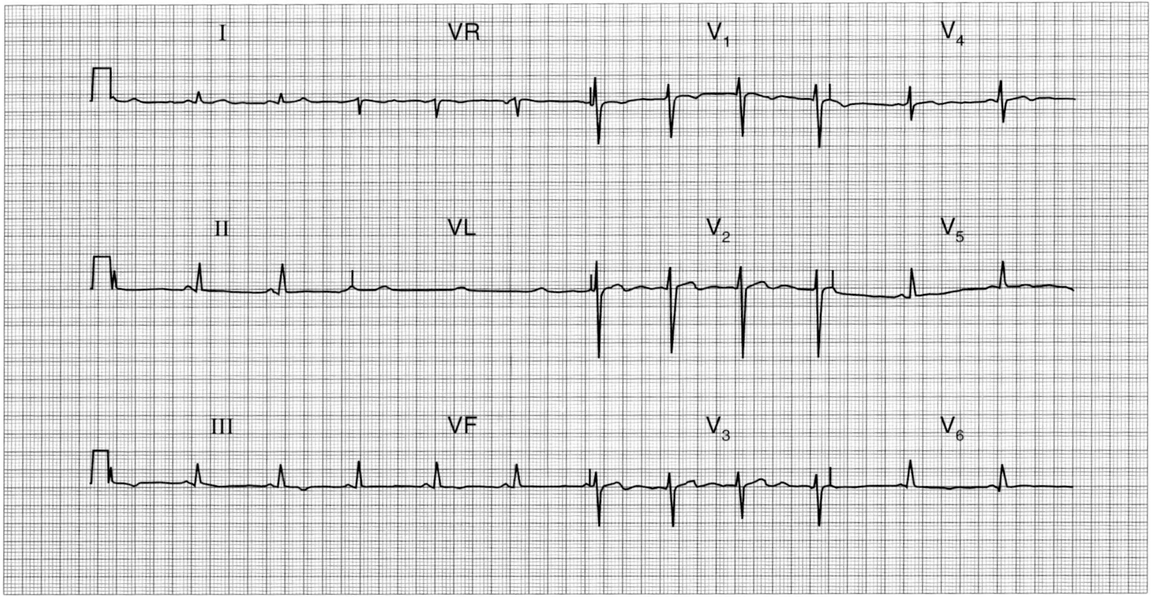

ECG 51 This ECG was recorded from a young man seen in the out-patient department with chest pain which appeared to be non-specific. How would you interpret the ECG and what action would you take?

ANSWER 51

The ECG shows:

- Sinus rhythm
- Normal axis
- Normal QRS complexes
- Inverted T waves in leads III, VF; biphasic T waves in lead V_4 and flattened T waves in leads V_5–V_6

Clinical interpretation

These T wave changes, particularly those in the inferior leads, could well be caused by ischaemia. The flattened T waves in the lateral leads can only be described as 'non-specific'.

What to do

When confronted with an ECG showing this sort of 'non-specific' abnormality, action depends primarily on the clinical diagnosis. If the patient is asymptomatic it is fair to report the ECG as showing 'non-specific changes'; if the patient has symptoms at all – as in this case – it is probably worth proceeding to an exercise test. In this patient, the exercise test was perfectly normal, and his symptoms cleared without any intervention. A repeat ECG, recorded purely out of interest a month later, showed similar changes.

Summary ★★★

Non-specific ST segment and T wave changes.

IP See p. 83

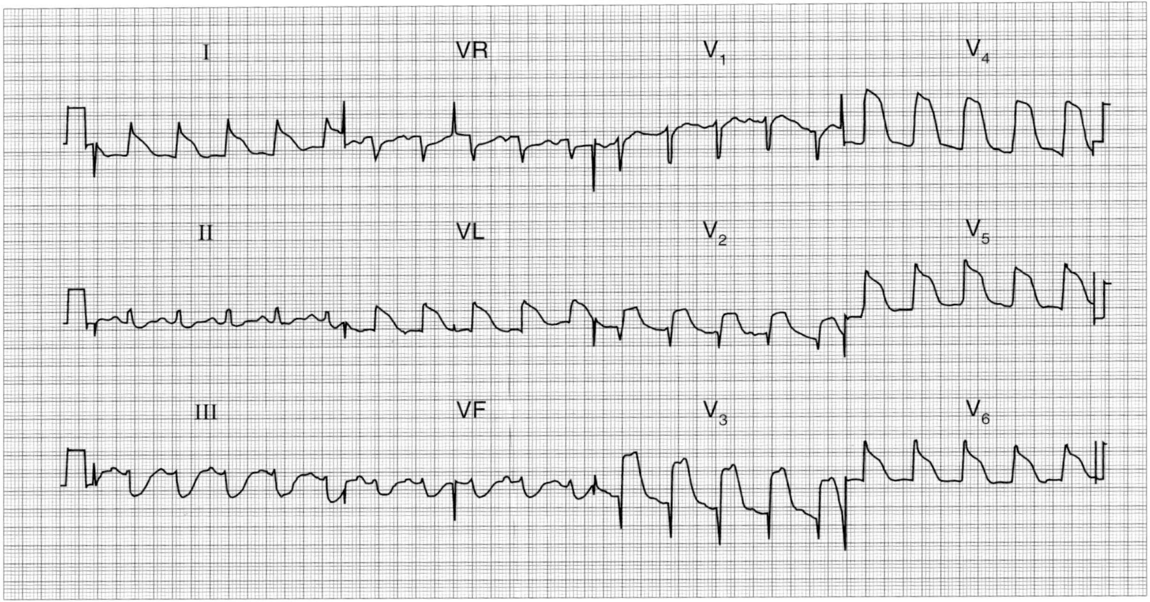

ECG 52 This ECG was recorded from a 65-year-old woman admitted to hospital as an emergency because of severe chest pain for 1 h. What does the ECG show? What other investigations would you order?

ANSWER 52

The ECG shows:

- Sinus rhythm
- Normal axis
- Probably normal QRS complexes
- Gross elevation of ST segments in anterior and lateral leads
- Depressed ST segments in the inferior leads and leads III, VF

Clinical interpretation
Acute anterolateral myocardial infarction. In the lateral leads I, VL and V_4–V_6, it is difficult to see where the QRS complexes end and the ST segments begin, but in lead II it is clear that the QRS complex is of normal width.

What to do
If the patient gives a history suggestive of a myocardial infarction and has this ECG, no further investigations are needed in the acute phase of the illness, and in particular there is no place for a chest X-ray. Routine treatment for a myocardial infarction – pain relief, aspirin and thrombolysis – should be commenced immediately.

Summary ★
Acute anterolateral myocardial infarction.

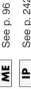

ME See p. 96
IP See p. 242

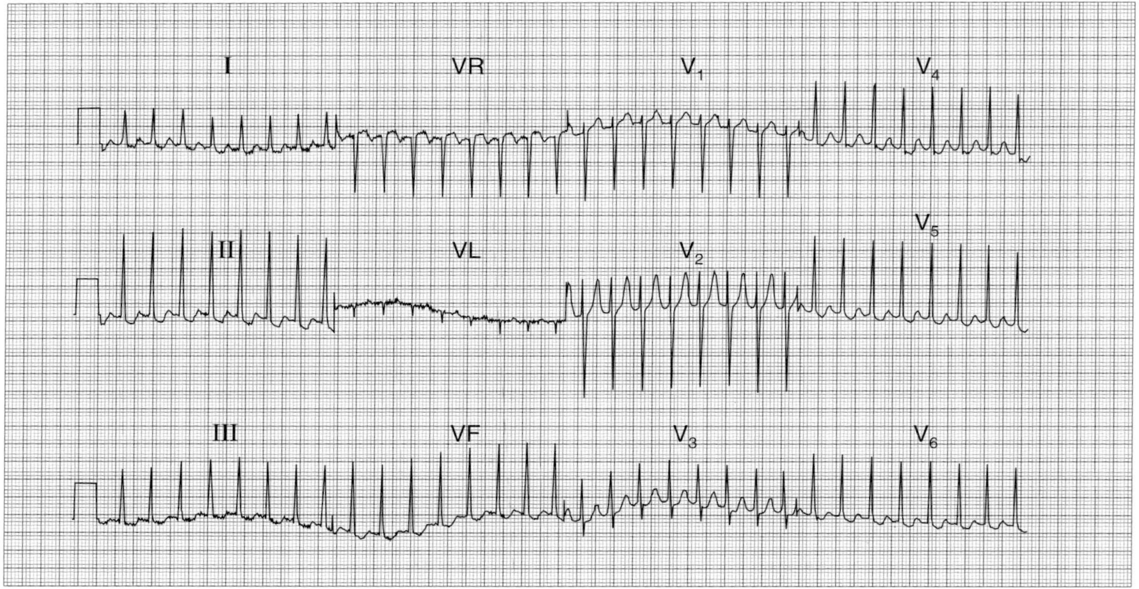

ECG 53 A 45-year-old woman had complained of occasional attacks of palpitations for 20 years, and eventually this ECG was recorded during an attack. What are the palpitations due to, and what would you do?

ANSWER 53

The ECG shows:

- Narrow complex tachycardia at 200/min
- No P waves visible
- Normal axis
- QRS complexes normal
- Some ST segment depression

Clinical interpretation

This ECG shows supraventricular tachycardia, probably junctional. These rhythms are usually due to a re-entry pathway within, or near to, the atrioventricular node. The ST segment depression could indicate ischaemia, but the ST segments are not horizontally depressed, nor is the depression greater than 2 mm, so it is probably of no significance.

What to do

The first action is carotid sinus pressure, which may terminate the attack. If this fails it will almost certainly respond to adenosine. As with any tachycardia, electrical cardioversion must be considered if there is haemodynamic compromise. Once sinus rhythm has been restored the patient must be taught the various methods (e.g. the Valsalva manoeuvre) with which she might try to terminate an attack. Prophylactic medication may not be needed if attacks are infrequent, but most patients with this problem should have an electrophysiological study to try to identify a re-entry pathway that can be ablated.

Summary ★
Supraventricular (junctional) tachycardia.

ME See p. 73
IP See pp. 29 and 167

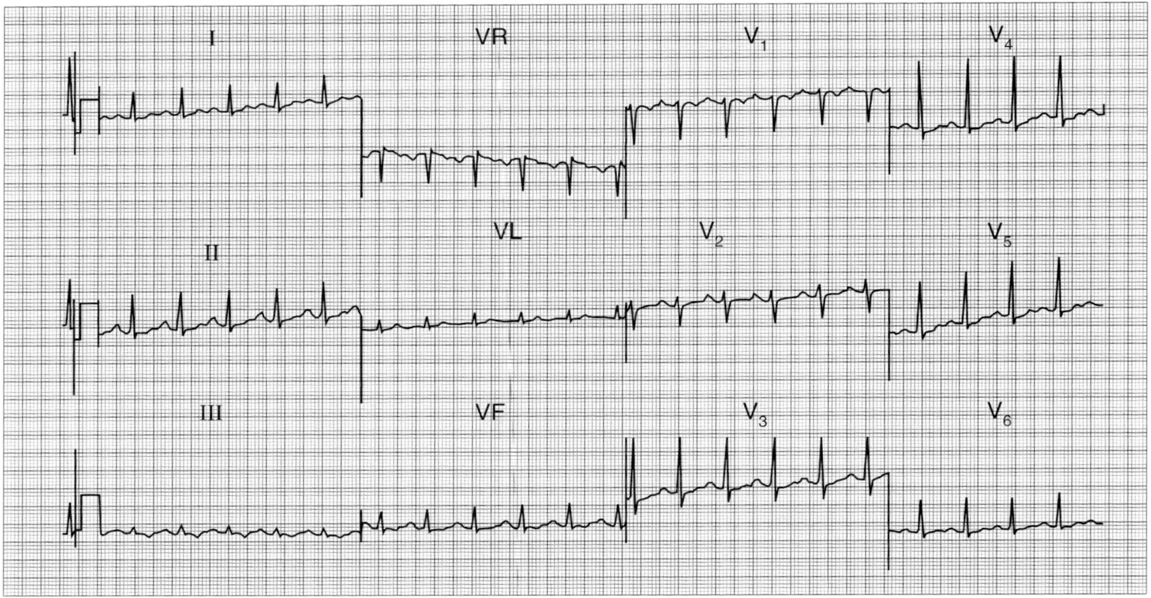

ECG 54 This ECG was recorded from a 35-year-old woman who complained of breathlessness. She was anxious, but there were no abnormalities on examination. Does this ECG help with her diagnosis and management?

ANSWER 54

The ECG shows:

- Sinus rhythm, rate 120/min
- Normal axis
- Normal QRS complexes
- Slight downward-sloping ST segment depression, especially in lead V_4
- Widespread T wave flattening
- T wave inversion in lead III

Clinical interpretation

A sinus tachycardia would be compatible with anxiety, though other causes of 'high output' (e.g. pregnancy, thyrotoxicosis, anaemia, volume loss, CO_2 retention, beri-beri) have to be considered. The widespread ST segment and T wave changes have to be described as 'non-specific'; in an anxious patient they could be due to hyperventilation. They do not help with diagnosis and management.

What to do

If a full history and examination fail to suggest any underlying physical disease, further investigations are unlikely to be helpful.

Summary ★★

Non-specific ST segment and T wave changes.

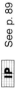

IP See p. 89

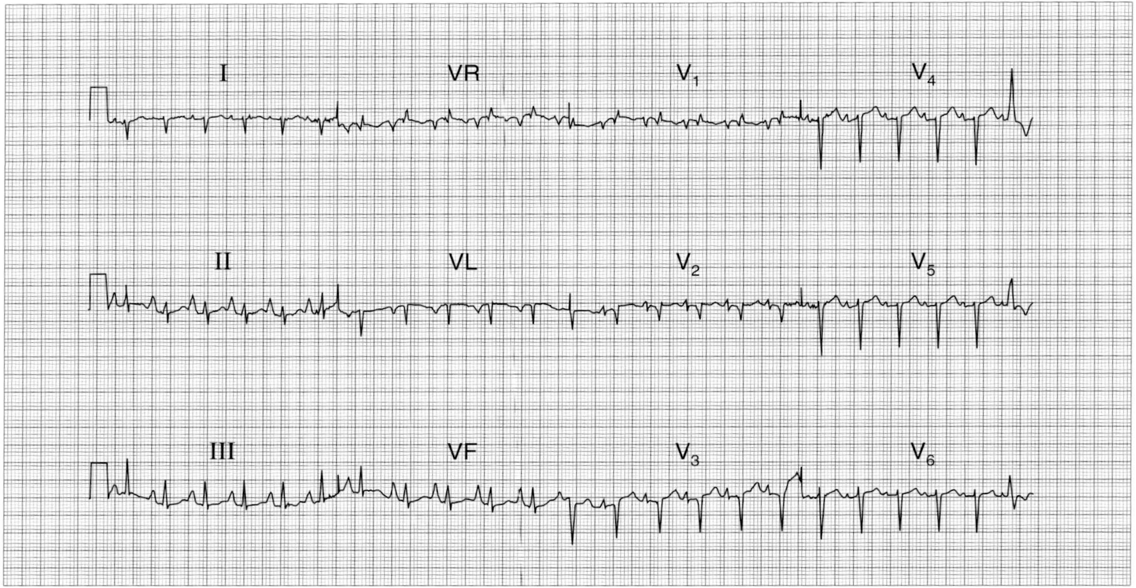

ECG 55 This ECG was recorded from a 60-year-old man seen in the clinic because of severe breathlessness, which had developed over several years. His jugular venous pressure is raised. What do you think the problem is?

ANSWER 55

The ECG shows:

- Sinus rhythm, rate 140/min
- One ventricular extrasystole
- Peaked P waves (best seen in leads II, III, VF)
- Normal PR interval
- Right axis
- Dominant R wave in lead V_1
- Deep S wave in lead V_6
- Normal ST segments and T waves

Clinical interpretation

The sinus tachycardia suggests a major problem. The peaked P waves indicate right atrial hypertrophy. The right axis and dominant R wave in lead V_1 suggest right ventricular hypertrophy. The deep S wave in lead V_6, with no 'left ventricular' complexes in the chest leads, indicates 'clockwise rotation' of the heart, with the right ventricle occupying the precordium. These changes suggest lung disease.

What to do

Since the ECG is entirely 'right sided' one can assume that the problem is due to chronic lung disease or recurrent pulmonary embolism.
The story sounds more in keeping with a lung problem. The raised jugular venous pressure is presumably due to cor pulmonale. The sinus tachycardia is worrying, and suggests respiratory failure.

Summary ★★

Sinus tachycardia and one ventricular extrasystole, right atrial and right ventricular hypertrophy, and clockwise rotation suggest chronic lung disease.

ME See pp. 64, 89 and 91

IP See p. 342

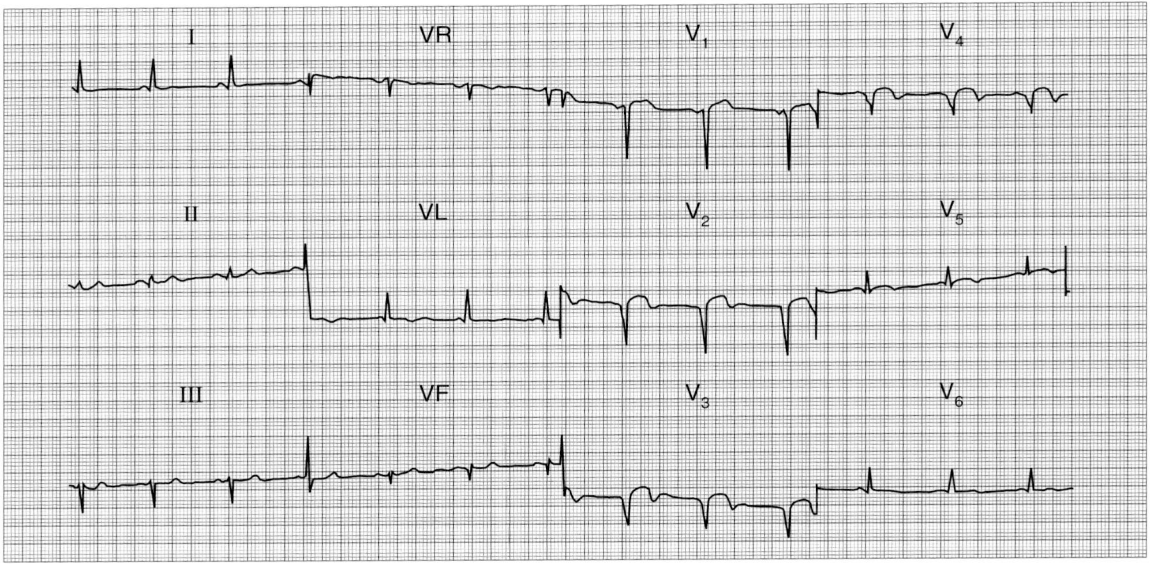

ECG 56 A 60-year-old man is seen in the out-patient department complaining of breathlessness which began quite suddenly 2 months previously. He had had no chest pain. Examination revealed a raised jugular venous pressure, basal crackles in the lungs and a third sound at the cardiac apex. This is his ECG. What does it show and how does it fit the clinical picture? What would you do?

ANSWER 56

The ECG shows:

- Sinus rhythm
- Normal axis
- Large Q waves in leads V_1–V_4 and small Q waves in leads I and VL
- Elevated ST segments and inverted T waves in leads V_2–V_5
- Flattened, biphasic T waves in leads I, VL, V_6

Clinical interpretation

This ECG would be compatible with an acute anterior myocardial infarction, but this does not fit the clinical picture: it appears that an event occurred 2 months previously. This pattern of ST segment elevation in the anterior leads can persist following a large infarction, and is seen in the presence of a ventricular aneurysm.

What to do

An echocardiogram will show if left ventricular function is impaired – which it almost certainly is – and if there is an aneurysm; an aneurysm was present in this case. The patient should be treated with diuretics and an angiotensin-converting enzyme inhibitor, and surgical resection of the aneurysm might be considered.

Summary ★★★
Old anterior myocardial infarction with a ventricular aneurysm.

ME See p. 95

IP See pp. 243, 250 and 314

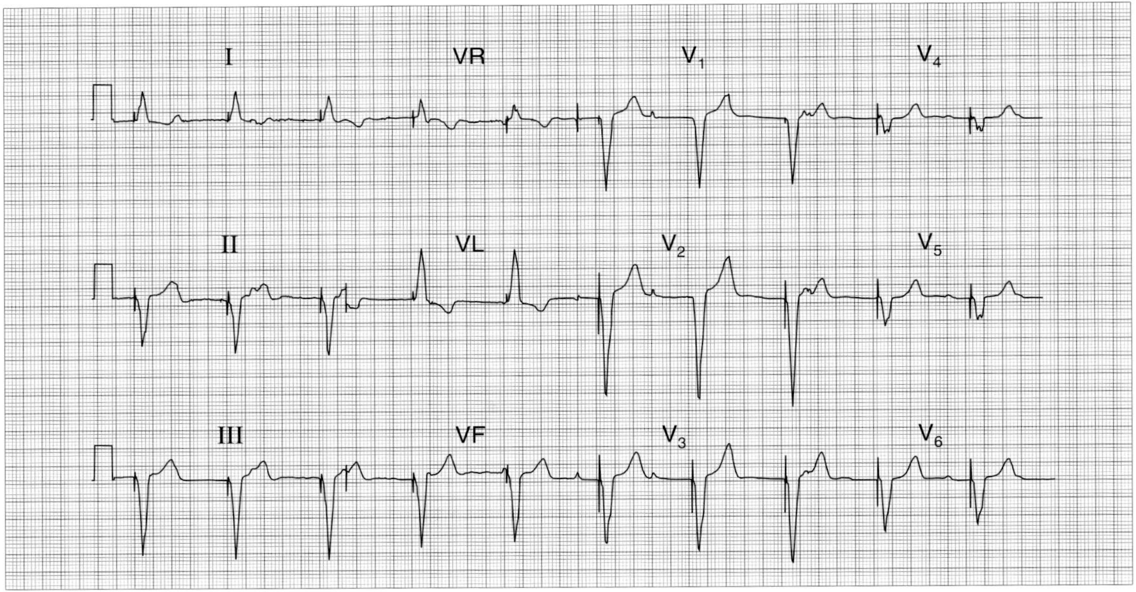

ECG 57 The senior house officer in the A & E department is puzzled by this ECG which was recorded from an 80-year-old admitted unconscious with a stroke. What has the house officer missed?

ANSWER 57

The ECG shows:

- Regular rhythm at 60/min
- Occasional P waves not related to QRS complexes (e.g. lead I)
- Left axis
- QRS complexes preceded by a sharp 'spike'
- Broad QRS complexes (160 ms)
- Deep S wave in lead V_6
- Inverted T waves in leads I and VL

Clinical interpretation

The broad QRS complexes show that this is either a supraventricular rhythm with bundle branch block, or a ventricular rhythm. This rhythm is ventricular. The sharp spikes preceding each QRS complex are due to a pacemaker. The P waves that can occasionally be seen indicate that the underlying rhythm, presumably the reason why the pacemaker was inserted, is complete heart block.

What to do

The SHO has missed the pacemaker, which is usually buried below the left clavicle. There is no particular reason why the pacemaker should be related to the stroke, except that patients with vascular disease in one territory usually have it in others – this man probably has both coronary and cerebrovascular disease.

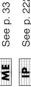

Summary ★
Permanent pacemaker and underlying compete block.

ME See p. 33
IP See p. 222

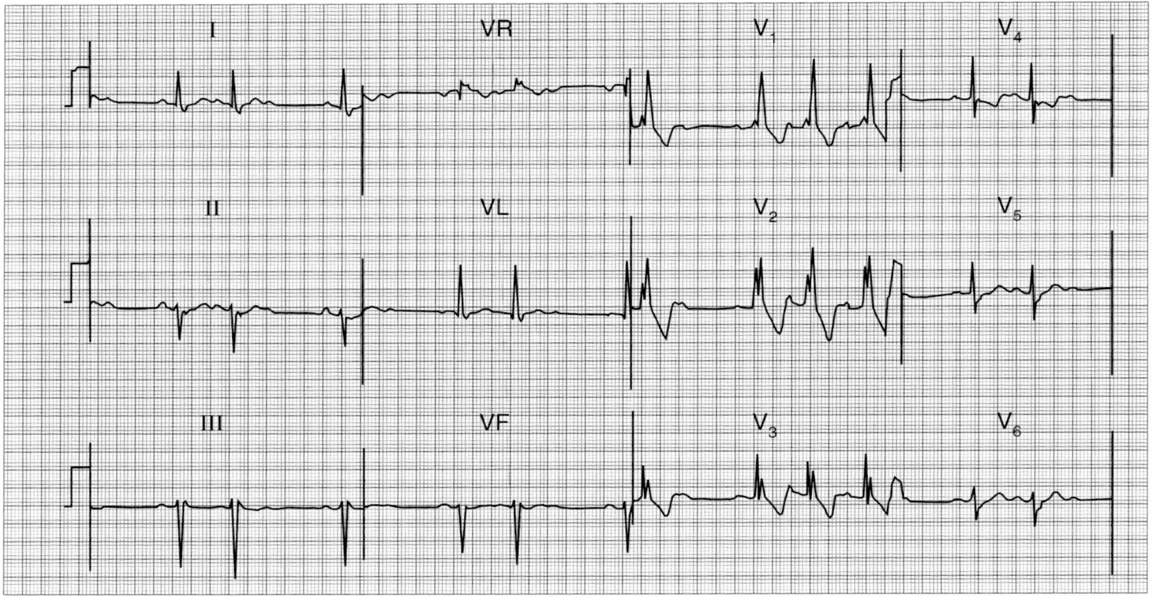

ECG 58 A 70-year-old woman who complained of 'dizzy turns' was found to have an irregular pulse, and this ECG was recorded. There are three abnormalities. What advice would you give her?

ANSWER 58

The ECG shows:

- Sinus rhythm
- Normal and constant PR intervals in the conducted beats
- Occasional non-conducted P waves
- Left axis deviation
- Right bundle branch block

Clinical interpretation

This combination of second degree block (Mobitz type 2) plus left axis deviation (left anterior hemiblock) with right bundle branch block indicates disease throughout the conduction system. This combination of conduction abnormalities is sometimes called 'trifascicular' block.

What to do

The 'dizzy turns' may represent intermittent complete block. Permanent pacing is essential.

Summary ★★

Second degree block (Mobitz type 2) and bifascicular block.

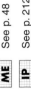

ME See p. 48

IP See p. 212

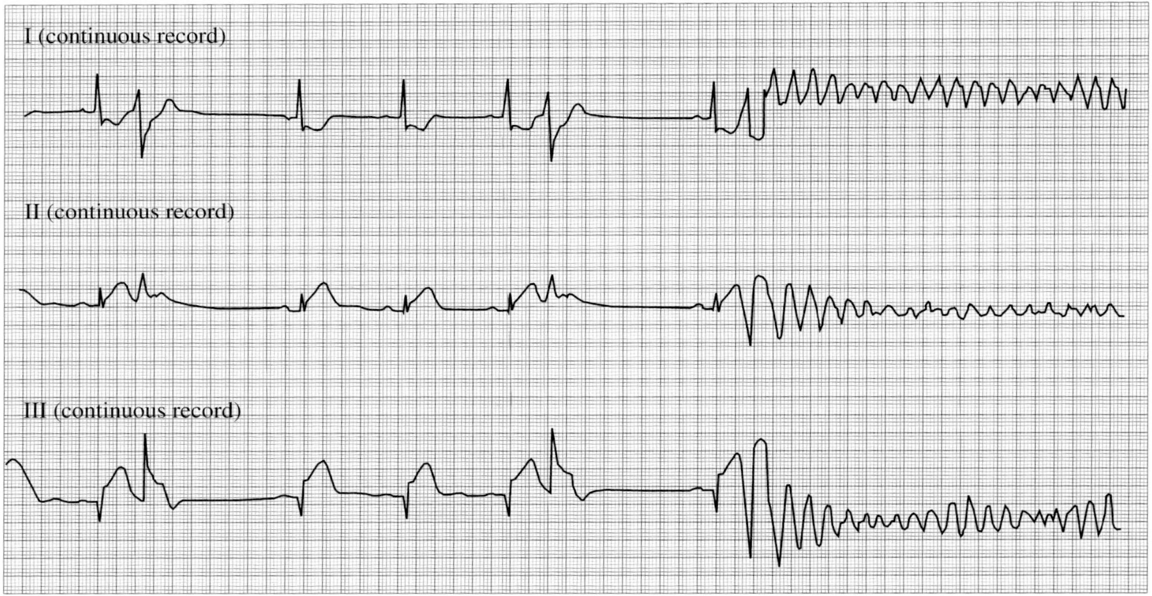

ECG 59 A 50-year-old man who had come to the A & E department with chest pain, collapsed while his ECG was being recorded. What happened and what would you do?

ANSWER 59

The ECG shows:

- Sinus rhythm with ventricular extrasystoles
- The third extrasystole occurs on the peak of the T of the preceding sinus beat
- After three or four beats of ventricular tachycardia ventricular fibrillation develops
- In the sinus beats there is a Q wave in lead III, raised ST segments in leads II and III, and ST segment depression and T wave inversion in lead I

Clinical interpretation

Although only leads I, II and III are available it looks as if the chest pain was due to an inferior myocardial infarction. This was probably the cause of the ventricular extrasystoles and an 'R on T' extrasystole caused ventricular tachycardia, which rapidly decayed the ventricular fibrillation. It might be argued that in lead III, and perhaps also in lead I, 'torsade de pointes' ventricular tachycardia is present, but this is not apparent in lead II.

What to do

Precordial thump and immediate defibrillation, but if no defibrillator is at hand then cardiopulmonary resuscitation should be performed, and the usual procedure for the management of the cardiac arrest instituted.

Summary ★
Probable inferior myocardial infarction; R on T ventricular extrasystole causing ventricular fibrillation.

ME See p. 80

IP See pp. 195 and 215

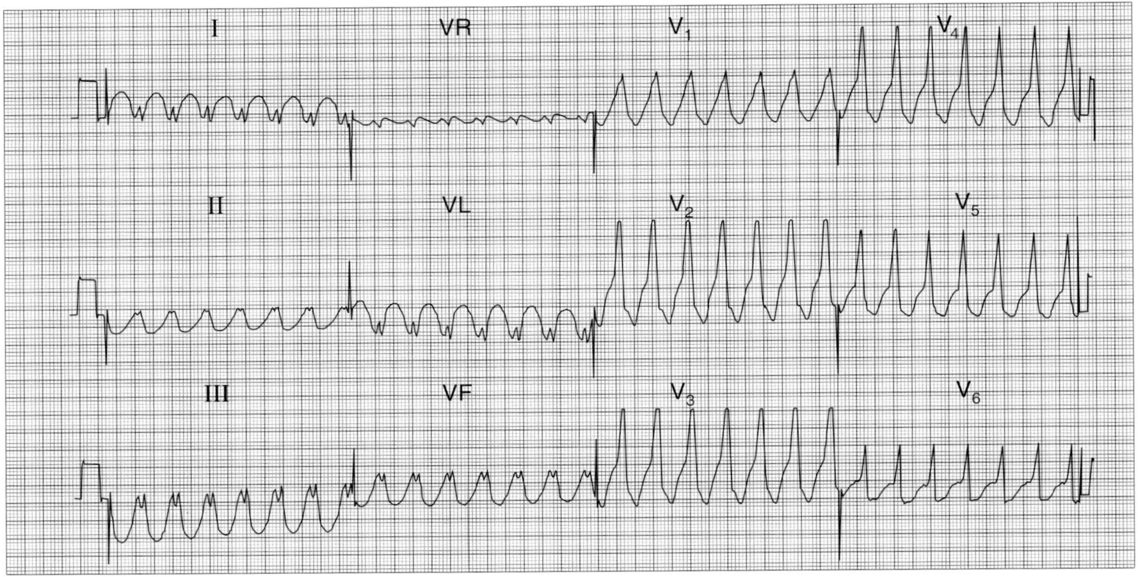

ECG 60 A 60-year-old man complained of severe central chest pain, and a few minutes later became extremely breathless and collapsed. He was brought to the A & E department where his heart rate was found to be 150/min, his blood pressure was unrecordable and he had signs of left ventricular failure. This is his ECG. What has happened and what would you do?

ANSWER 60

The ECG shows:

- Broad complex tachycardia at 150/min
- No P waves visible
- Normal axis
- QRS duration about 200 ms
- Concordance of QRS complexes (i.e. all point upwards) in the chest leads

Clinical interpretation

A broad complex tachycardia can be ventricular in origin, or can be due to a supraventricular tachycardia with aberrant conduction (i.e. bundle branch block). Here the very broad complexes and the QRS concordance suggest a ventricular tachycardia. In a patient with a myocardial infarction it is always safe to assume that such a rhythm is ventricular. From the story, one would guess that this patient had a myocardial infarction and then developed ventricular tachycardia, but it is possible that the chest pain was due to the arrhythmia.

What to do

This patient has haemodynamic compromise – low blood pressure and heart failure – and needs immediate cardioversion. While preparations are being made it would be reasonable to try intravenous lignocaine or amiodarone.

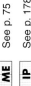

Summary ★

Ventricular tachycardia.

ME See p. 75

IP See p. 178

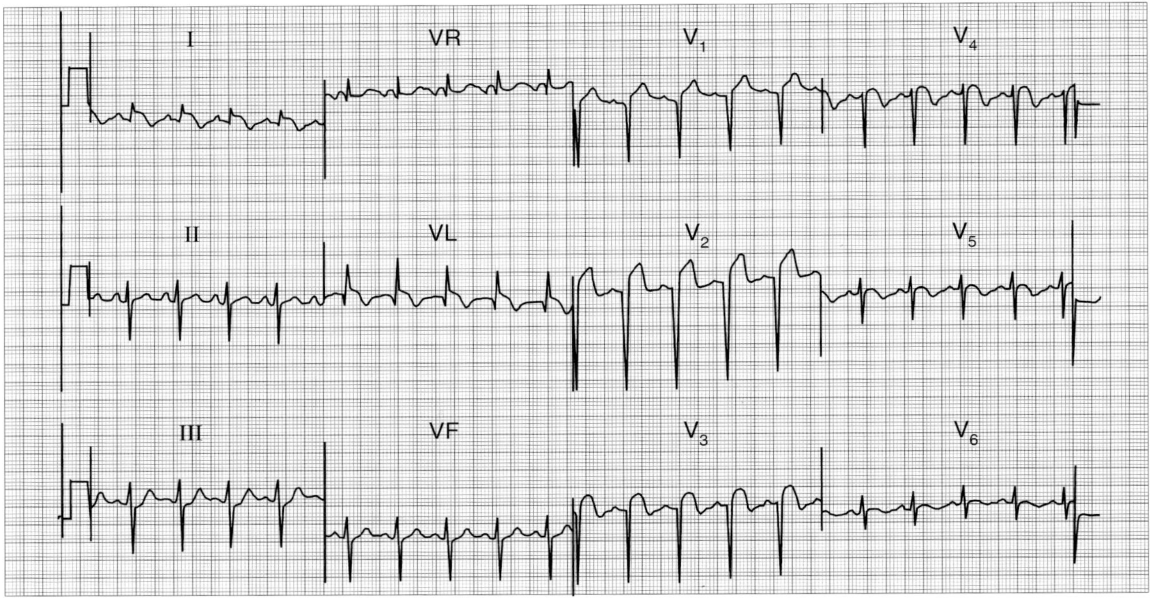

ECG 61 A 70-year-old man who gave a history of several years of chest pain on exertion, and of breathlessness, was admitted to hospital with severe central chest pain. This is his ECG. What does it show? What physical signs would you expect to find?

ANSWER 61

The ECG shows:

- Sinus rhythm
- Left axis deviation
- Q wave in lead VL; QS pattern in leads V_2–V_3
- Persistent S waves in lead V_5
- Raised ST segments and inverted T waves in leads V_1, VL
- Raised ST segments in leads V_2–V_3 with biphasic T waves in leads V_3–V_4

Clinical interpretation

Left axis deviation is due to left anterior hemiblock, probably associated with the infarction shown in the anterior leads: it is difficult to be sure of the age of this infarction. The ECG appears to show an acute lateral infarction. The persistent S waves in lead V_6 suggest chronic lung disease.

What to do

The patient has probably had quite severe left ventricular damage and may have the signs of left ventricular failure; he may well also have signs of chronic airway disease.

Summary ★★★

Acute lateral myocardial infarction, anterior infarction of uncertain age, left axis deviation and possible chronic lung disease.

ME See p. 98

IP See pp. 242 and 342

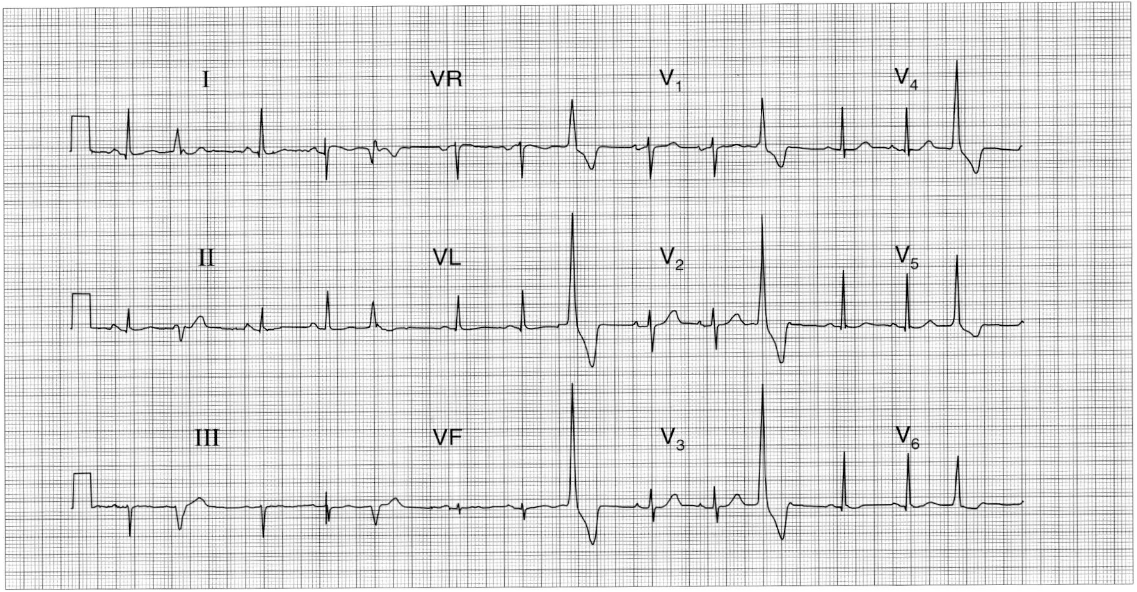

ECG 62 This ECG was recorded from a 30-year-old woman who complained of an irregular heart beat, especially on lying down at night. She is worried about heart disease. What would you advise her to do?

ANSWER 62

The ECG shows:

- Sinus rhythm, rate 85/min
- Frequent ventricular extrasystoles
- Normal axis in sinus beats
- Sinus beats show normal QRS complexes, ST segments and T waves

Clinical interpretation

This ECG is normal apart from the ventricular extrasystoles. Provided there is nothing else in the history or physical examination to suggest heart disease, the extrasystoles are not important.

What to do

The patient must be reassured that extrasystoles do not of themselves indicate heart disease.
She should be advised not to smoke, and to try abstaining from alcohol, coffee and tea to see if the extrasystoles become less troublesome. Medication is best avoided, but if she insists on treatment a beta-blocker will be safe.

Summary ★
Normal ECG with ventricular extrasystoles.

ME See p. 64
IP See p. 155

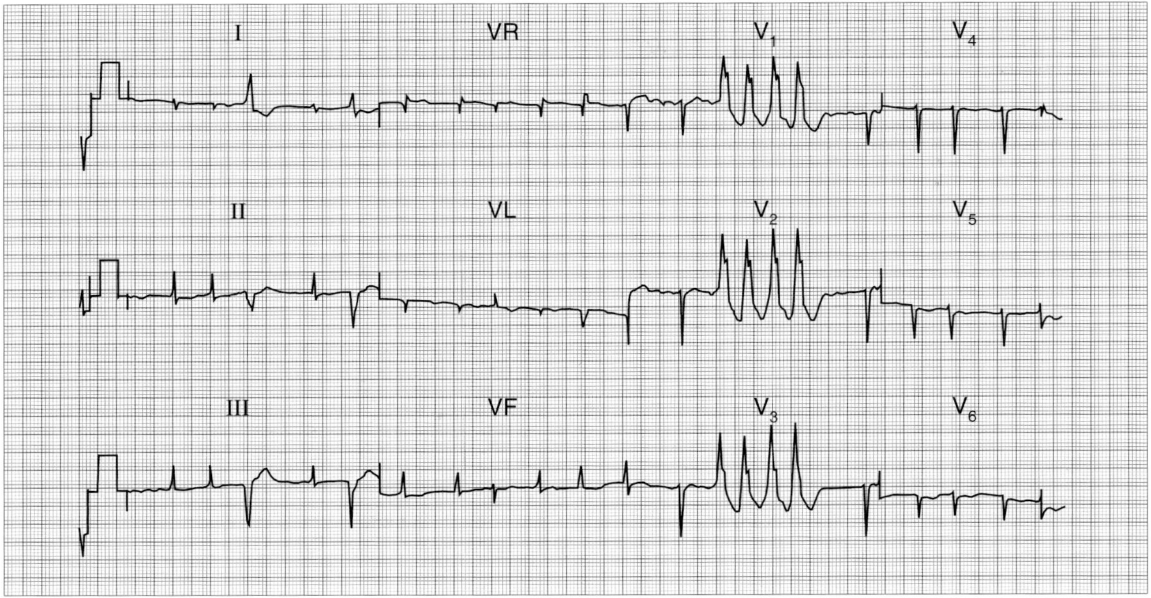

ECG 63 A 60-year-old man who was being treated in hospital complained of palpitations, and this ECG was recorded. What do you think the underlying disease was, and what were the palpitations due to?

ANSWER 63

The ECG shows:

- Atrial fibrillation
- Ventricular extrasystoles with two distinct morphologies (best seen in lead II)
- A four-beat run of ventricular tachycardia
- Right axis deviation
- Small QRS complexes
- No R wave development in the chest leads; lead V_6 shows a dominant S wave
- T wave inversion in leads V_5, V_6

Clinical interpretation

This ECG suggests chronic lung disease – small complexes, right axis deviation, and marked 'clockwise rotation' with lead V_6 still showing a ight ventricular type of complex. The atrial fibrillation is probably secondary to the lung disease, though the usual other possibilities must be considered. The patient's lung condition is probably being treated with a beta-agonist, such as salbutamol, and this could be the cause of the extrasystoles and ventricular tachycardia.

What to do

Stop the beta-agonist but do not give a beta-blocker. Check the electrolyte levels; consider the possibility of digoxin toxicity.

Summary ★★★

Atrial fibrillation with ventricular extrasystoles and ventricular tachycardia; changes suggesting chronic lung disease.

ME See pp. 64, 75 and 78

IP See pp. 170, 175 and 178

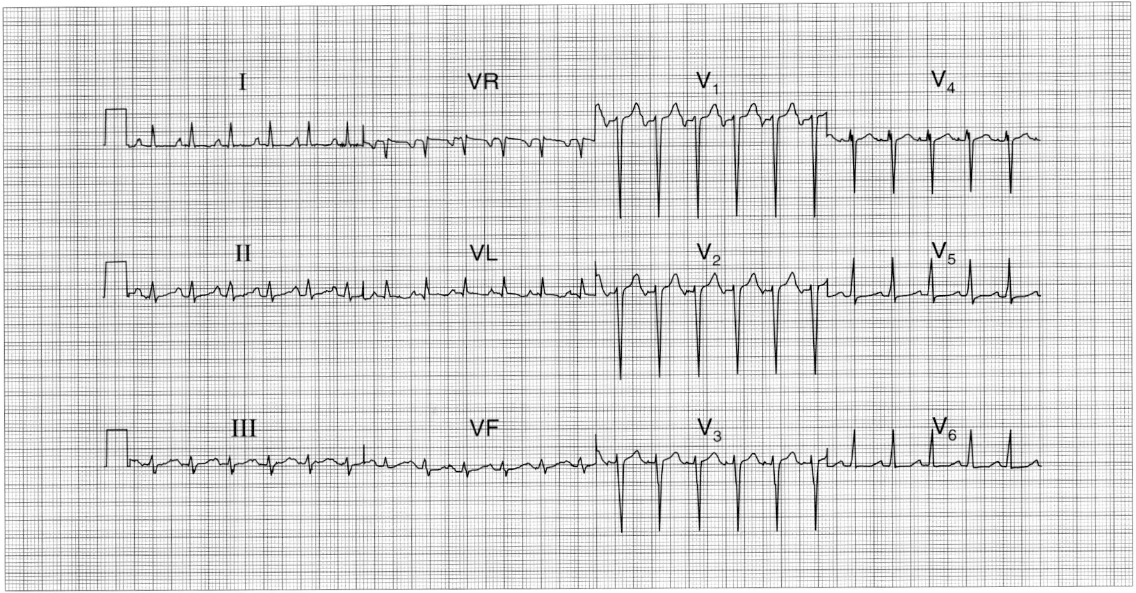

ECG 64 A 45-year-old man complained of palpitations, weight loss and anxiety. His blood pressure was 180/110, and his heart seemed normal. This is his ECG. His thyroid function tests, measured several times, were normal. What might be going on?

ANSWER 64

The ECG shows:

- Narrow complex rhythm at 140/minute
- Apparently one P wave per QRS complex
- Normal PR interval
- Normal axis
- Normal QRS complexes
- Inverted T wave in lead VL and a flat T wave in leads I, V_5–V_6

Clinical interpretation

The immediate problem is to decide whether this is a sinus or atrial tachycardia. Carotid sinus pressure caused transient slowing, so this is probably sinus rhythm. A sinus tachycardia of 140/min could be due to anxiety, but seems very fast for this; other possibilities are drug effects (beta-agonists, amphetamine) and a phaeochromocytoma – which turned out to be the diagnosis.

Summary ★★
Sinus tachycardia.

ME See p. 54

IP See p. 152

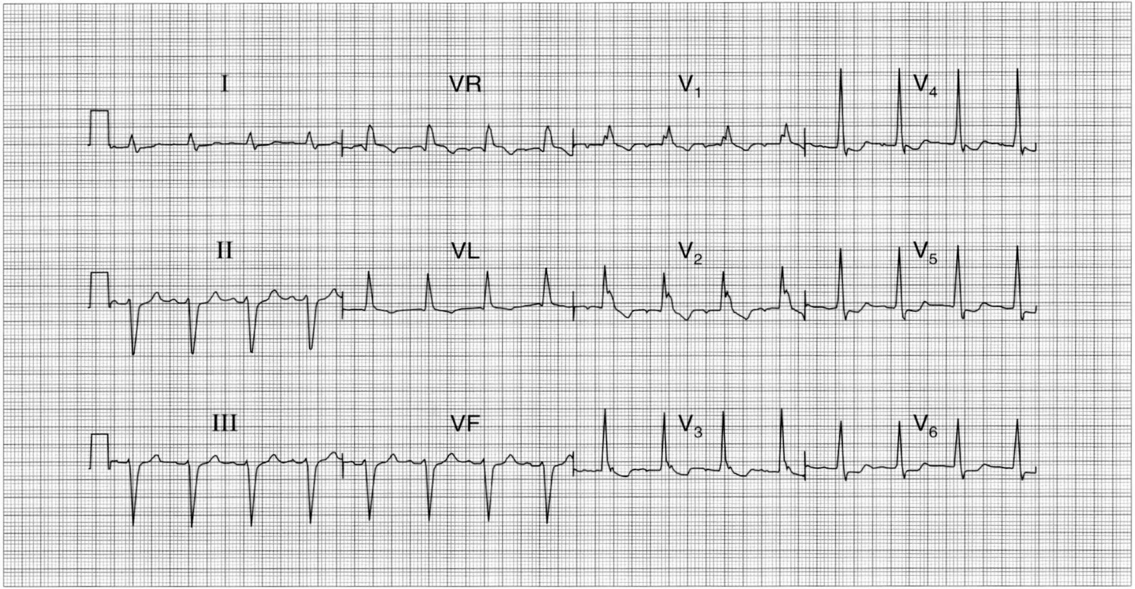

ECG 65 A 70-year-old man is sent to the clinic because of rather vague dizzy attacks, which occur approximately once per week. Otherwise he is well, and there are no abnormalities on examination. Does this ECG help with his management?

ANSWER 65

The ECG shows:

- Sinus rhythm, rate 100/min
- PR interval at the upper limit of normal (200 ms)
- Left axis
- QRS duration prolonged (160 ms)
- RSR pattern in lead VL, wide S wave in lead V_6
- Inverted T waves in leads VL, V_1–V_4

Clinical interpretation

The left axis is accompanied by widening of the QRS complexes and an inverted T wave in lead VL, and this is characteristic of left anterior hemiblock. There is also right bundle branch block, so two of the main conducting pathways are blocked, which is known as 'bifascicular block'. The fact that the PR interval is at the upper limit of normal raises the possibility of delayed conduction in the remaining pathway; if the PR interval were definitely prolonged the pattern would be called 'trifascicular block'.

What to do

Bifascicular block is not an indication for pacing if the patient is asymptomatic. The problem here is to decide if the dizzy attacks are due to intermittent complete heart block. Ideally an ECG would be recorded during an attack; since they only occur every week or so, ambulatory ECG tape recording may not be helpful, but an event recorder would be worth trying. In the absence of clear evidence the decision whether or not to insert a permanent pacemaker is a matter of judgement, but in a patient with this story and ECG it would be a perfectly reasonable thing to do.

Summary ★★

Left anterior hemiblock and right bundle branch block – bifasciular block.

ME See p. 48

IP See pp. 141 and 147

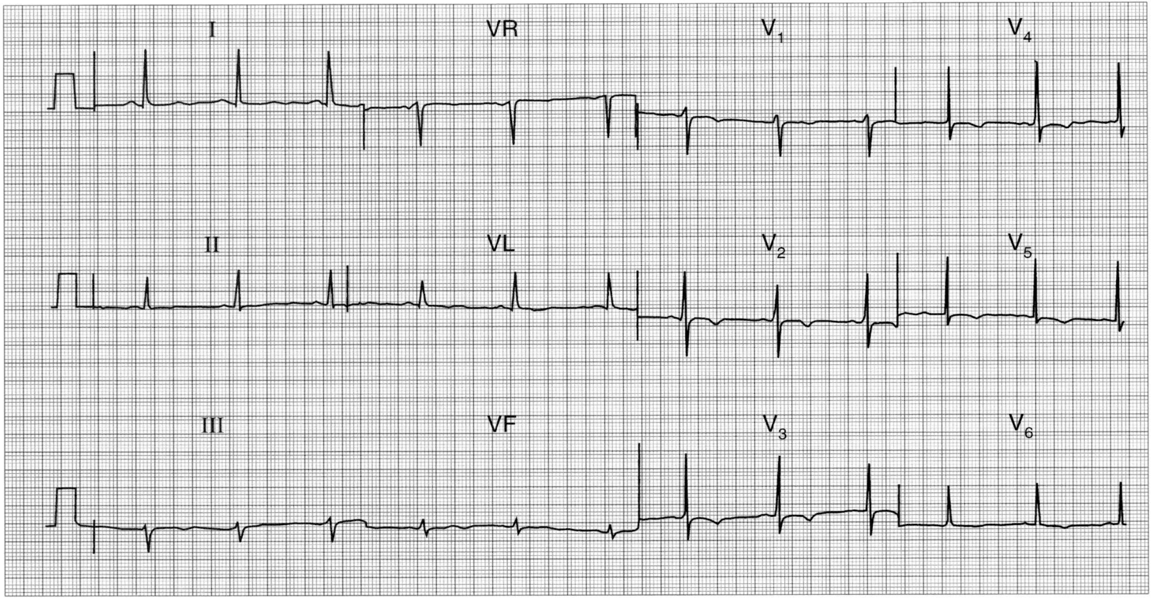

ECG 66 This ECG was recorded from a 25-year-old black football professional. What does it show, and what would you do?

ANSWER 66

The ECG shows:

- Sinus rhythm
- Normal axis
- Normal QRS complexes
- Widespread T wave inversion, particularly in leads V_2–V_5

Clinical interpretation

Repolarization (T wave) abnormalities are quite common in black people, but alternative explanations for this ECG appearance would be a non-Q wave infarction, or a cardiomyopathy.

What to do

This man is a professional football player, so it is important to exclude hypertrophic cardiomyopathy, and this can be done by echocardiography. Because his career depended upon coronary disease being excluded, a coronary angiogram was performed and was entirely normal.

Summary ★★★
Widespread T wave inversion, probably normal in a black man.

ME See p. 112

IP See pp. 91 and 117

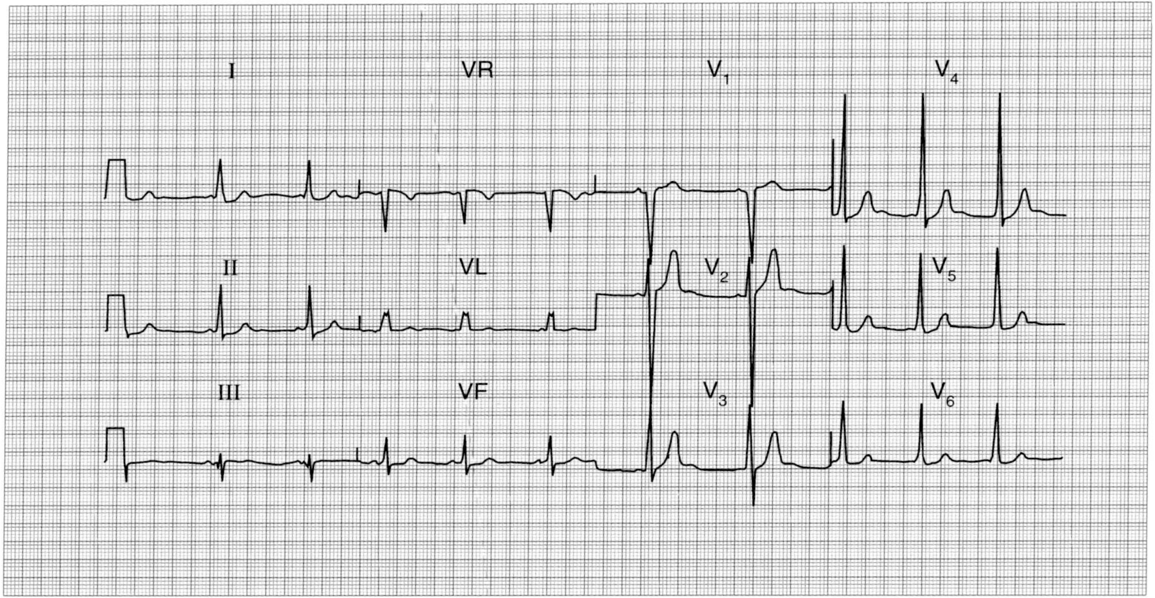

ECG 67 This ECG was recorded from an asymptomatic 20-year-old man at a pre-employment medical examination. The employer will require him to hold a vocational (HGV) driving licence. What advice would you give?

ANSWER 67

The ECG shows:

- Sinus rhythm
- Very short PR interval
- Normal axis
- Widened QRS complexes with a slurred upstroke (delta wave), best seen in leads I and V_4

Clinical interpretation

This is the Wolff–Parkinson–White syndrome: the accessory pathway is on the right side and this is sometimes called 'type B'.

What to do

It would be prudent to obtain an echocardiogram to make sure there is no structural abnormality (such as a cardiomyopathy) as well as the Wolff–Parkinson–White syndrome. Provided there is no history to suggest an arrhythmia, he can hold a vocational driving licence.

Summary ★★
Wolff–Parkinson–White syndrome.

ME See p. 81

IP See pp. 38 and 120

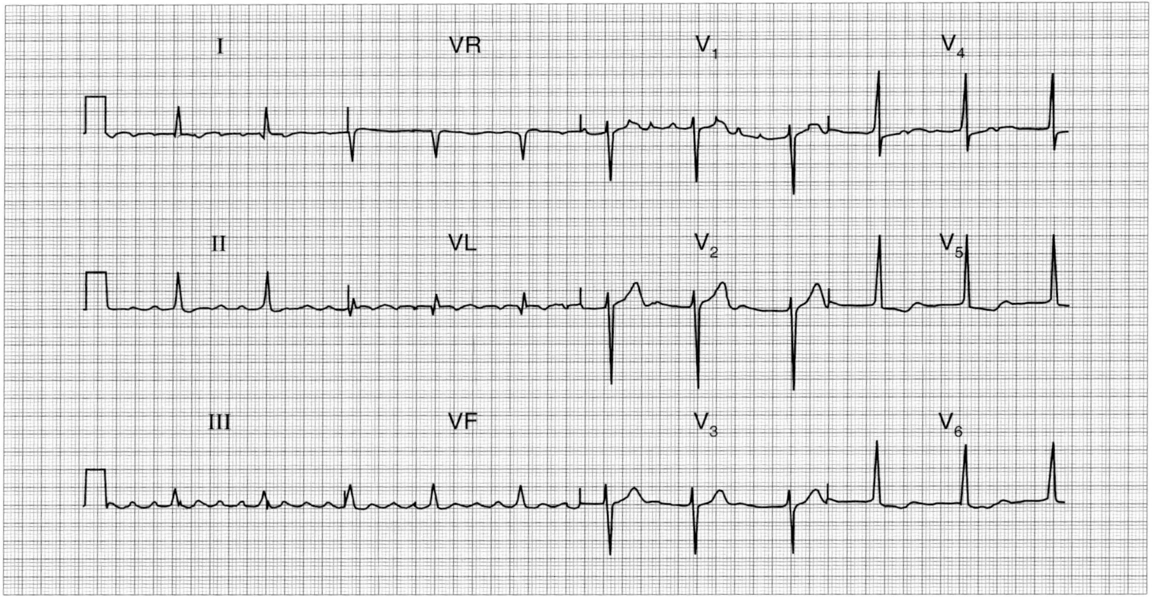

ECG 68 A 60-year-old woman is seen in the out-patient department complaining of breathlessness. There are no abnormal physical findings. What does this ECG show, what might be the underlying problem, and how would you treat her?

ANSWER 68

The ECG shows:

- Atrial flutter
- 4:1 block
- Normal axis
- Normal QRS complexes
- Sloping ST segment depression, best seen in leads V_5–V_6

Clinical interpretation

This shows atrial flutter with what appears to be a stable 4:1 block. The ST segment depression suggests digoxin effect.

What to do

The stable 4:1 block has caused a regular heart beat, so the arrhythmia was not suspected at the time of the clinical examination. There is nothing in this ECG to indicate the underlying disease, which could be ischaemic, rheumatic or a cardiomyopathy; echocardiography is needed. Digoxin will tend to maintain a fairly high degree of block but will not affect the underlying rhythm. Intravenous flecainide may convert the heart to sinus rhythm, but DC cardioversion may be necessary.

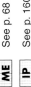

Summary ★★
Atrial flutter with 4:1 block.

ME See p. 68
IP See p. 160

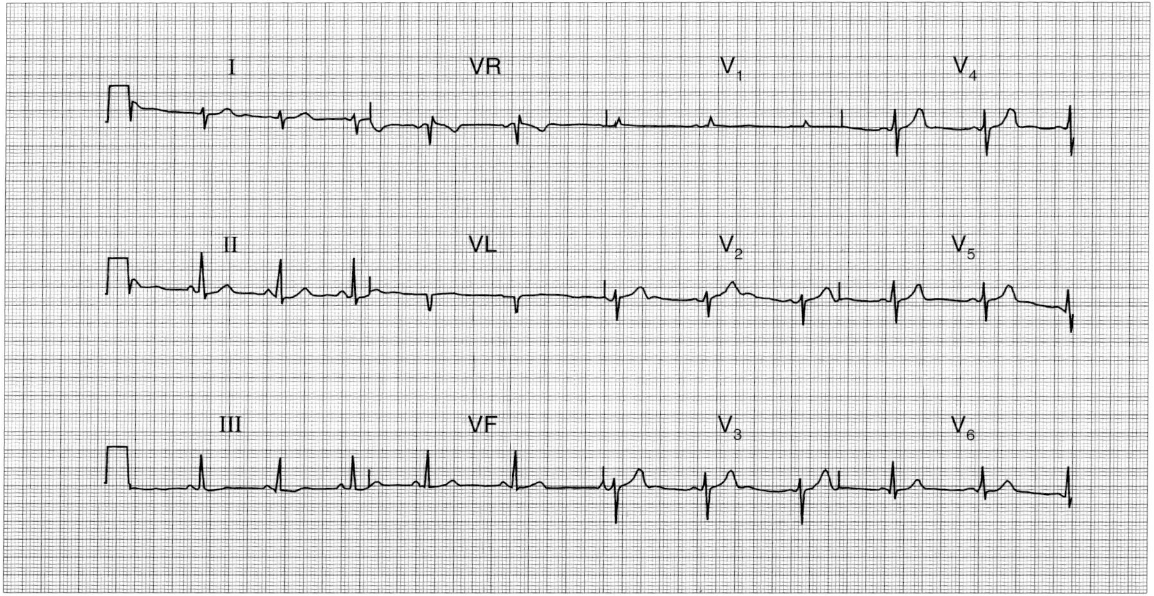

ECG 69 This ECG was recorded from a 30-year-old man at a medical examination required by the Civil Aviation Authority. Is it normal?

ANSWER 69

The ECG shows:

- Sinus rhythm
- Right axis deviation (dominant S waves in lead I)
- Dominant R wave in lead V_1
- Prominent U waves in leads V_2–V_5

Clinical interpretation

Right axis deviation can be a normal variant (particularly in tall thin people) but also occurs with right ventricular hypertrophy. The small dominant R wave in lead V_1 suggests right ventricular hypertrophy, but this can be a normal variant. The U waves could indicate hypokalaemia, but when associated with normal T waves (as here) they are a normal variant.

What to do

Exclude causes of right ventricular hypertrophy. A chest X-ray with a lateral view, and an echocardiogram will help determine whether the right ventricle really is enlarged.

Summary ★★★
Probably a normal ECG.

ME See p. 22

IP See pp. 69 and 74

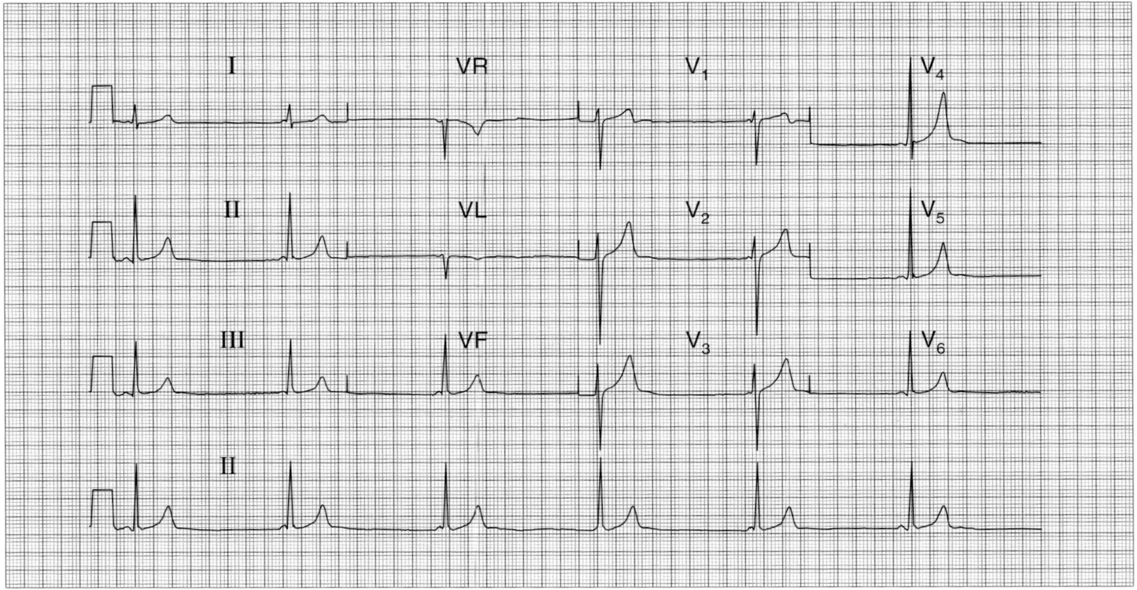

ECG 70 This ECG was recorded as part of the 'screening' examination of a young professional football player. Is it normal?

ANSWER 70

The ECG shows:

- Regular narrow complex rhythm at 35/min
- P waves sometimes, but not always, visible just before the QRS complexes
- PR interval, when measurable, is always short but varies
- Height of R wave in lead V_4 plus depth of S wave in lead V_2 = 45 mm
- Normal QRS complexes and ST segments.
- Peaked T waves, especially in lead V_4

Clinical interpretation

The short PR interval raises the possibility of pre-excitation, but the interval varies, and in the first complex of leads V_1–V_3 no P wave can be seen. The slow, narrow, complex rhythm suggests atrioventricular nodal escape. Here there is a pronounced slowing of the sinoatrial node, presumably due to athletic training, and an accelerated idionodal rhythm has taken over. This pattern used to be called a 'wandering atrial pacemaker'. The tall R waves are perfectly normal in young fit people, and so are the peaked P waves.

What to do

This is a normal variant in athletes, and no action is required.

Summary ★★
Accelerated idionodal rhythm.

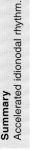

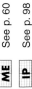

ME See p. 60

IP See p. 98

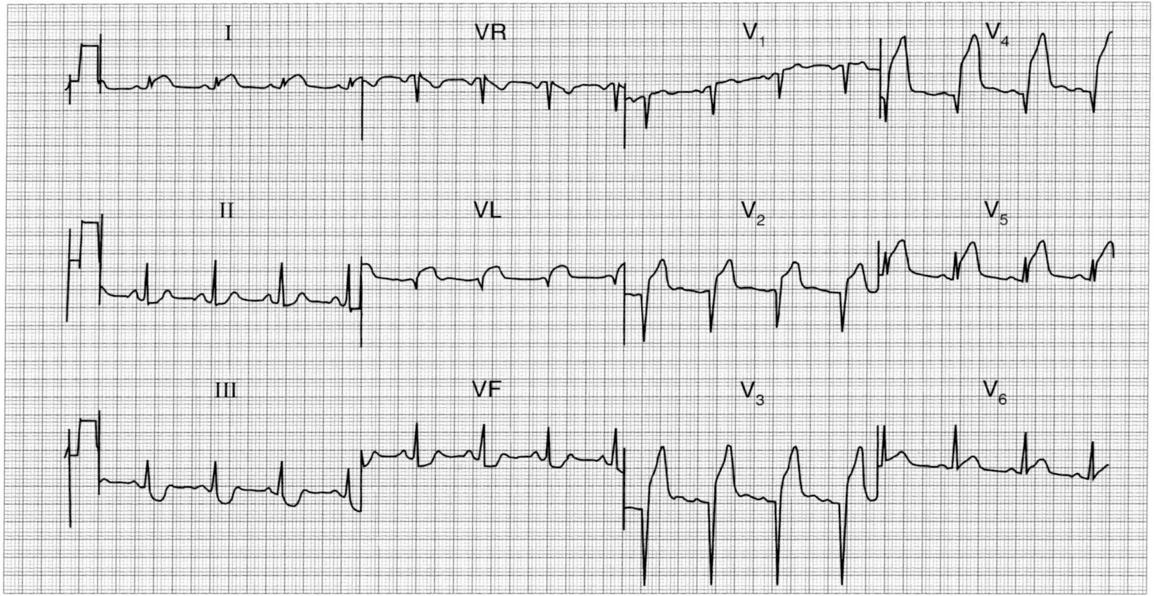

ECG 71 A 45-year-old patient is admitted to the A & E department having had severe central chest pain for 1 h. There are no signs of heart failure, and this is his ECG. What does the ECG show and what would you do?

ANSWER 71

The ECG shows:

- Sinus rhythm
- Normal axis
- Q waves in leads V_2–V_4
- Raised ST segments in leads I, VL, V_2–V_5
- Flat ST segment depression in leads III, VF

Clinical interpretation
This ECG shows an acute anterior myocardial infarction with inferior ischaemia.

What to do
Unless there are any potential risks of bleeding (previous stroke, peptic ulcer, diabetic retinopathy, etc.) this patient should be given aspirin, 300 mg to be chewed, and then a thrombolytic agent. The choice of agent is still open to debate: since he has not had a thrombolytic agent before, the cheaper agent streptokinase would be perfectly acceptable, but there is some evidence that the more expensive alteplase (rt-PA) reduces mortality more effectively, perhaps especially in young patients with anterior infarcts.

Summary ★
Acute anterior myocardial infarction and inferior ischaemia.

ME See p. 95
IP See p. 242

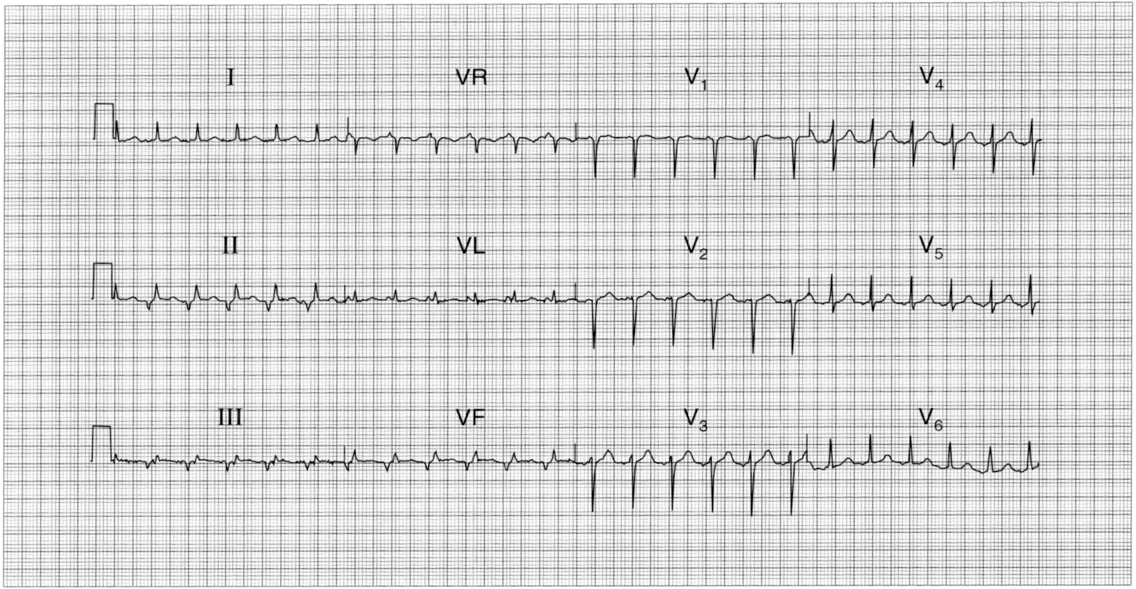

ECG 72 A 30-year-old man, who had complained of palpitations for many years without anything abnormal being found, came to the A & E department during an attack, and this ECG was recorded. Apart from signs of marked anxiety there was nothing to find except a heart rate of 140/min. What does the ECG show?

ANSWER 72

The ECG shows:

- Narrow complex tachycardia at 140/min
- Inverted P waves, most obvious in leads II, III, VF
- Short PR interval (about 100 ms)
- Normal axis
- Normal QRS complexes, ST segments and T waves

Clinical interpretation

The story of attacks of palpitations could indicate episodes of sinus tachycardia due to anxiety, but the heart rate of 140/min suggests a rhythm other than sinus rhythm is likely. This ECG clearly shows a supraventricular tachycardia of some sort, with one P wave per QRS complex. It could be sinus tachycardia, and the short PR interval could indicate pre-excitation, but the abnormal P waves in the inferior leads show that this is an atrial tachycardia.

What to do

Carotid sinus massage may terminate the attack, but if not it will almost certainly respond to adenosine. Further attacks may be prevented by a beta-blocker, but the patient should be referred for an electrophysiological study in the hope that a re-entry pathway can be identified and ablated.

Summary ★★

Atrial tachycardia.

ME See p. 67

IP See p. 159

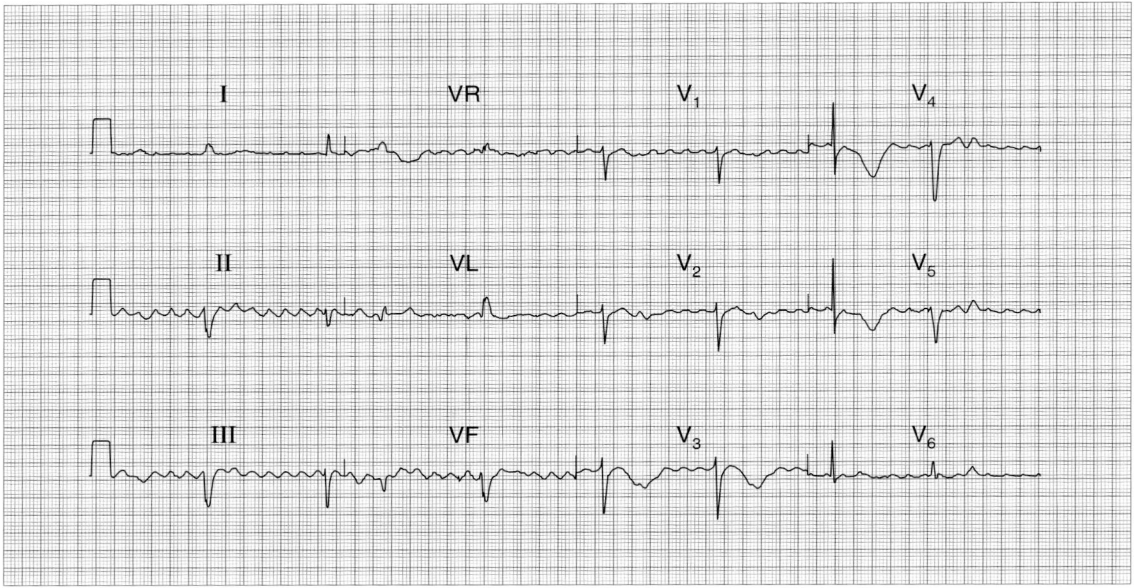

ECG 73 A confused 80-year-old woman was sent in from a nursing home because of a collapse. No other history was available, except that she was said to be having treatment for her heart. There were no obvious physical signs, but this is her ECG. What is going on?

ANSWER 73

The ECG shows:

- Atrial flutter with a ventricular rate of 50/min
- Ventricular extrasystoles
- Left axis
- Normal QRS complexes
- Inverted T waves in the anterior leads
- Prolonged QT interval (about 650 ms)

Clinical interpretation

The atrial flutter with a slow ventricular rate raises the possibility that a bradycardia caused her collapse; the left anterior hemiblock indicates that she has conduction tissue disease. The anterior T wave inversion may be due to ischaemia. There is no ST segment depression, suggesting that she is taking digoxin, but the prolonged QT interval suggests either an electrolyte abnormality or that she is being treated with one of the many drugs that have this effect. A collapse in a patient with a long QT interval suggests torsade de pointes ventricular tachycardia. Since she has atrial flutter you need to think about amiodarone – which is what she turned out to be taking.

Summary ★★★
Atrial flutter with a slow ventricular rate, ventricular extrasystoles, left anterior hemiblock and a prolonged QT interval.

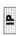

IP See pp. 375 and 376

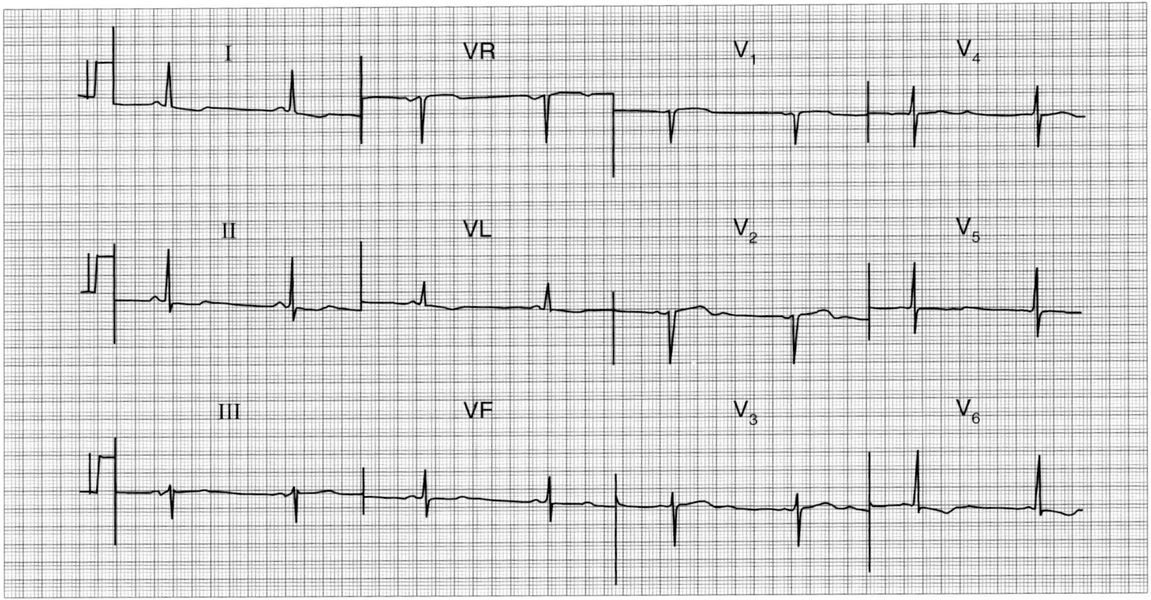

ECG 74 This ECG was recorded as part of a routine health check on a 50-year-old woman who said she was asymptomatic. The only other abnormality detected in the usual screening tests was a serum cholesterol level of 7.2 mmol/l. What would you do?

ANSWER 74

The ECG shows:

- Sinus rhythm
- Normal axis
- Normal QRS complexes
- Widespread T wave flattening and inversion
- Prominent U waves especially V_3–V_5

Clinical interpretation

Flattened T waves with prominent U waves usually result from hypokalaemia. The serum potassium level is usually checked during health screening, but the same ECG changes can result from hypocalcaemia or hypomagnasaemia. A high cholesterol level can be a marker for coronary disease, but elevated cholesterol levels can also be secondary to thyroid or renal disease.

What to do

Check the thyroid function. This woman had myxoedema, and her ECG became normal when it was treated.

Summary ★★★
Widespread T wave flattening with prominent U waves – classically due to hypokalaemia, but in this case due to myxoedema.

ME See p. 108

IP See pp. 362 and 368

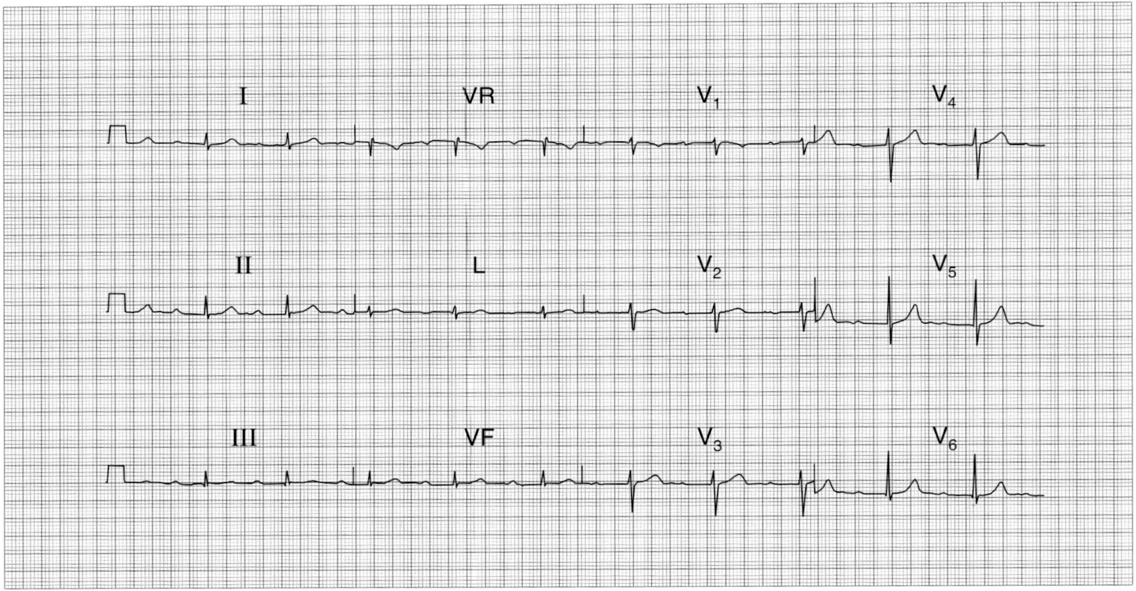

ECG 75 This ECG was recorded from an asymptomatic 45-year-old man at a 'health screening' examination. Is it normal, and what advice would you give him?

ANSWER 75

The ECG shows:

- Sinus rhythm, rate 64/min
- Prolonged PR interval (360 ms)
- Normal QRS complexes, ST segments, and T waves

Clinical interpretation

This ECG shows first degree atrioventricular block but is otherwise entirely normal.

What to do

Although the upper limit of the PR interval is usually taken to be 200 ms, longer durations (technically first degree block) are frequently seen in healthy people. Provided you can be sure that this patient has no symptoms, and provided the physical examination is normal, no further action is required. Some individuals in occupations that require a totally normal ECG may have to have an ambulatory ECG recording to demonstrate that there are no episodes of higher-degree block.

Summary ★
First degree atrioventricular block.

ME See p. 30

IP See pp. 62 and 137

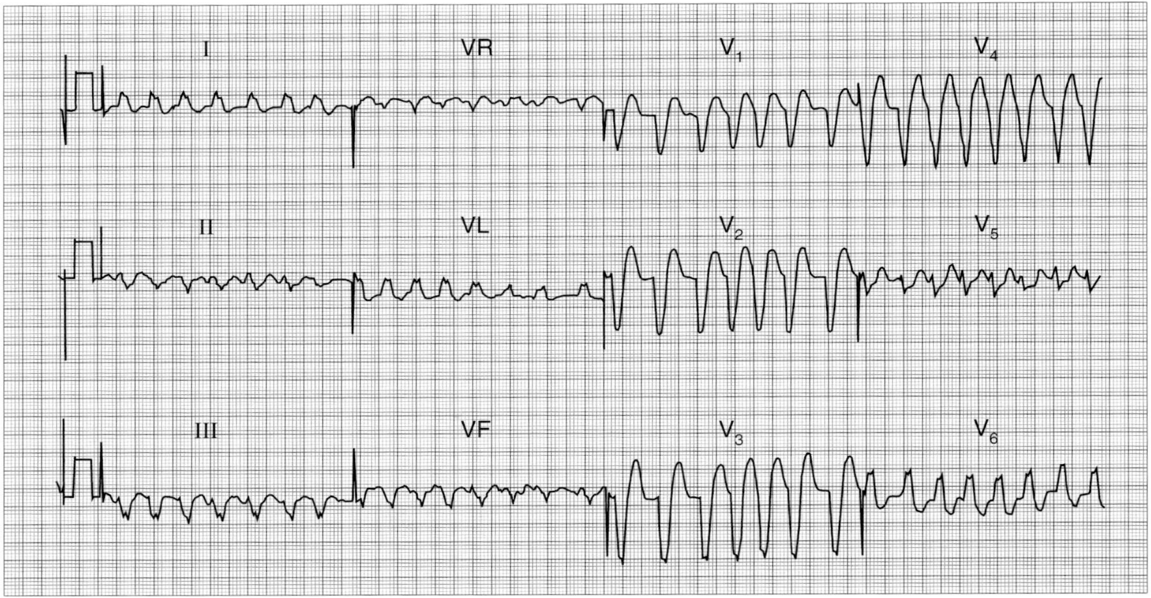

ECG 76 An 80-year-old woman was admitted to hospital because of a sudden onset of palpitations associated with breathlessness. She was in congestive cardiac failure and had a heart murmur suggestive of aortic stenosis. What does this ECG show and how would you treat her?

ANSWER 76

The ECG shows:

- Broad-complex tachycardia
- Irregular rhythm, rate 130–200/min
- No clear P waves but irregular baseline, best seen in lead VL
- Left bundle branch block pattern

Clinical interpretation

The marked irregularity of rhythm, coupled with the irregular baseline glimpsed in one beat in lead VL, shows that this is atrial fibrillation with left bundle branch block.

What to do

Aortic stenosis is commonly associated with left bundle branch block. In the presence of aortic stenosis, vasodilators must be used with caution and she should be treated with digoxin and diuretics. As soon as possible the aortic valve gradient should be assessed by echocardiography, and even at the age of 80 years, aortic valve replacement might be considered.

Summary ★★

Atrial fibrillation with left bundle branch block.

ME See pp. 36 and 78

IP See p. 117

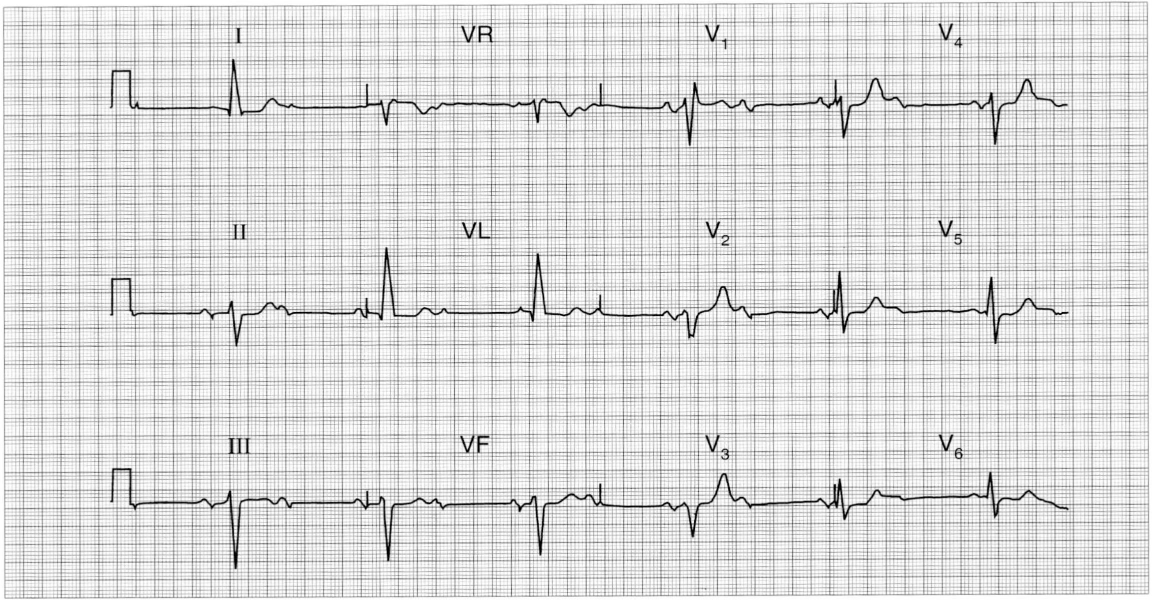

ECG 77 An 80-year-old man is found at routine examination to have a slow heart rate and a harsh systolic murmur. This is his ECG. What does it show, and what is the likely diagnosis? Is treatment necessary?

ANSWER 77

The ECG shows:

- Sinus rhythm, P wave rate 75/min
- Second degree (2:1) block
- Left axis deviation
- Right bundle branch block

Clinical interpretation

This is second degree block and not complete (third degree) block because the PR interval in the conducted beats is normal: at times it appears to vary but in fact this variation is due to lead changes. Left axis deviation (left anterior hemiblock) and right bundle branch block constitute bifascicular block, but the 2:1 block shows that there is also disease either in the His bundle or in the remaining posterior fascicle. This combination is sometimes called 'trifascicular' block.

What to do

The combination of a heart murmur and heart block suggests aortic stenosis. The severity of this can be assessed with echocardiography, though the slow rate (and thus high stroke volume) will accentuate the recorded valve gradient. Aortic valve replacement may or may not be needed, but the patient certainly needs a permanent pacemaker to prolong his survival.

Summary ★★
Second degree (2:1) block and bifascicular block.

ME See pp. 32 and 48

IP See pp. 141 and 146

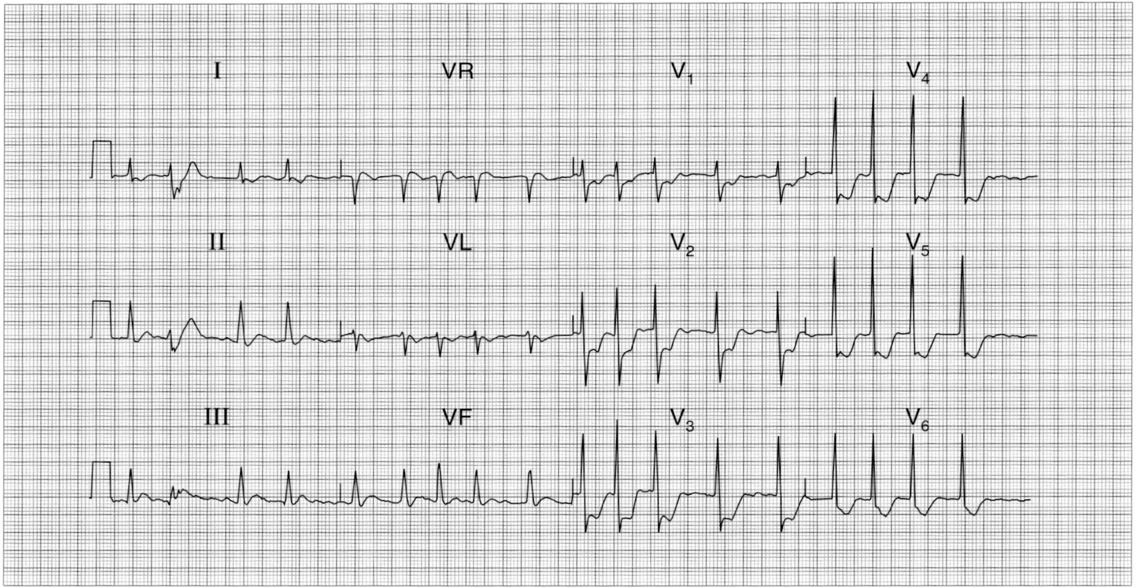

ECG 78 A 70-year-old woman, who had been breathless for several months, was admitted with chest pain, and this is her ECG. What does it show and what would you do?

ANSWER 78

The ECG shows:

- Atrial fibrillation with one ventricular extrasystole
- Ventricular rate about 110/min
- Normal axis
- Normal QRS complexes
- Horizontal ST segment depression of up to 7 mm in leads V_2–V_5
- Downward-sloping ST segment depression in lead V_6
- Inverted T waves in leads I, VL, V_6, and indeterminate T waves elsewhere

Clinical interpretation

The anterior horizontal ST depression indicates severe ischaemia, which is presumably the cause of the chest pain. The downward-sloping ST segment in lead V_6 could be due to digoxin therapy. The ventricular rate is not too fast, and although the heart rate may be contributing to the ishchaemia it seems unlikely that it is the main problem.

What to do

The patient should be treated for an acute coronary syndrome with heparin, a beta-blocker and nitrates. If the pain does not settle, early angiography with a view to revascularization by a coronary artery bypass graft (CABG) or percutaneous transluminal angioplasty (PTCA) will have to be considered.

Summary ★★
Atrial fibrillation and anterior ischaemia.

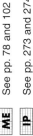

ME See pp. 78 and 102

IP See pp. 273 and 274

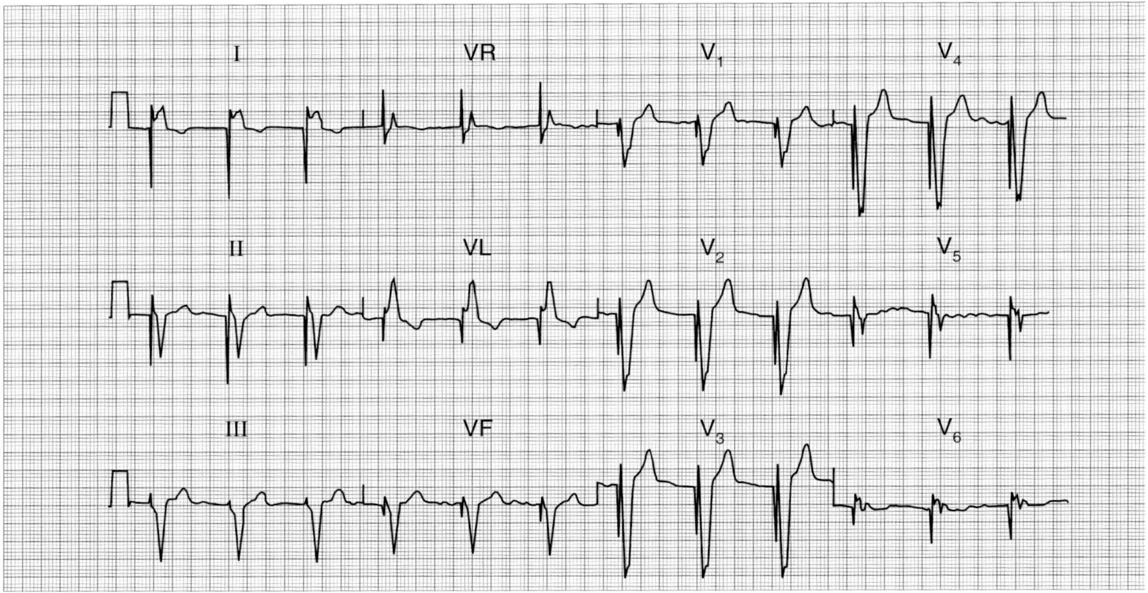

ECG 79 An elderly woman is admitted to hospital unconscious, evidently having had a stroke. No cardiac abnormalities are noted, but this is her ECG. What has been missed?

ANSWER 79

The ECG shows:

- No P waves; irregular baseline suggesting atrial fibrillation
- Regular QRS complexes
- Left axis deviation
- Wide QRS complexes of an indeterminate pattern
- Each QRS complex is preceded by a deep and narrow spike

Clinical interpretation

The narrow spike is due to a pacemaker, and someone has not noticed the permanent pacing battery which is probably below the left clavicle. The pacing wire will be stimulating the right ventricle, giving rise to broad QRS complexes resembling a bundle branch block pattern. The underlying rhythm here is atrial fibrillation: the patient may have had atrial fibrillation with complete block, or there may simply have been a slow ventricular response to the atrial fibrillation.

What to do

The stroke may have been due to an embolus arising in the left heart as a result of atrial fibrillation. There may have been temporary pacemaker failure, but probably the stroke was not related to the pacemaker.

Summary ★★

Ventricular-paced rhythm and atrial fibrillation.

IP See p. 222

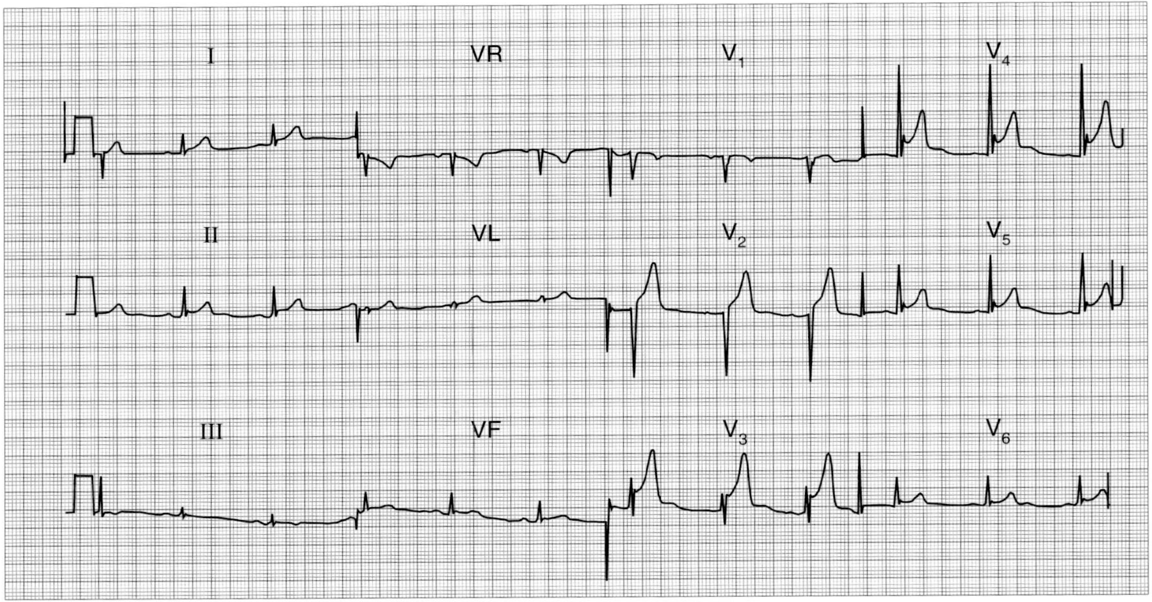

ECG 80 A 30-year-old man is seen in the A & E department with left-sided chest pain that appears to be pleuritic in nature. What does his ECG show?

ANSWER 80

The ECG shows:

- Sinus rhythm
- Normal axis
- Normal QRS complexes
- Raised ST segments in leads II, V_3–V_6, in each case preceded by an S wave

Clinical interpretation

When a raised ST segment follows an S wave as shown here, it is called 'high take-off' of the ST segment. This is a normal variant, which must be distinguished from the changes associated with an acute infarction or pericarditis.

What to do

If the patient has chest pain that appears to be pleuritic, then pulmonary rather than cardiac causes of pain should be considered – infection, pulmonary embolus and pneumothorax. The ECG is completely unhelpful here.

Summary ★★

Normal ECG showing 'high take-off' ST segment.

IP See pp. 82 and 84

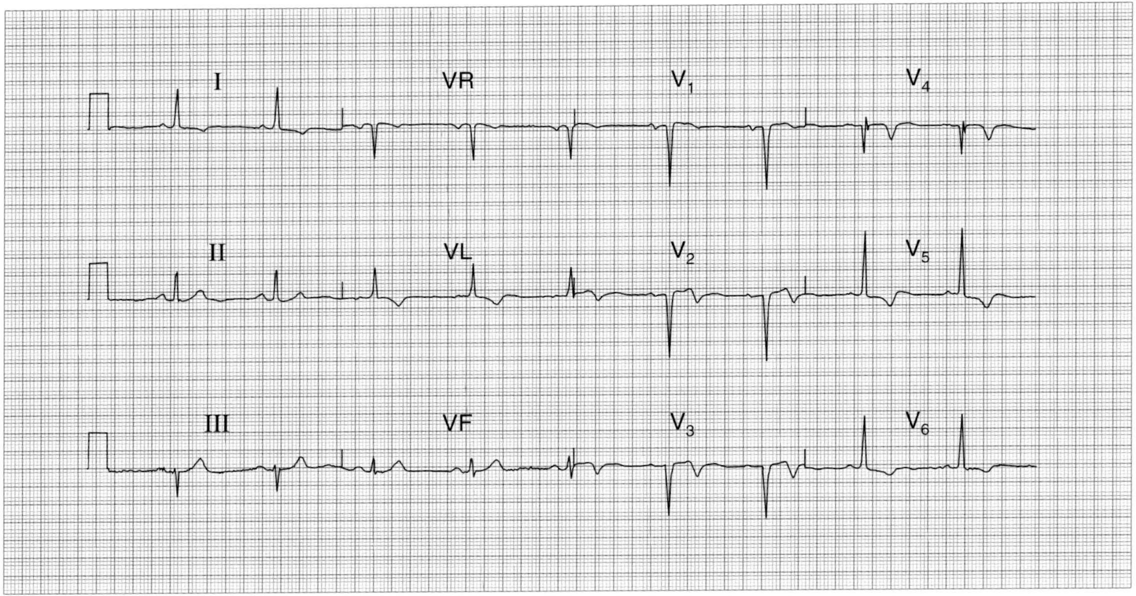

ECG 81 A 50-year-old man returned from holiday in Spain saying that while there he had had some bad indigestion, but was now perfectly well. This is his ECG: what does it show and what would you do?

ANSWER 81

The ECG shows:

- Sinus rhythm
- Normal conduction
- Normal axis
- Q waves in leads V_2–V_4
- Slightly elevated ST segments in leads V_2–V_3
- Inverted T waves in leads I, VL, V_2–V_6

Clinical interpretation

This ECG shows an old anterior myocardial infarction with lateral ischaemia. The slight elevation of ST segments might suggest an acute process if the pain were recent, but with this story the changes are almost certainly old.

What to do

The assumption has to be that the 'indigestion' was actually a myocardial infarction. Since he is now well, the important thing is to ensure that he takes the appropriate steps to prevent a further attack – he must stop smoking and reduce weight if necessary, and he should be treated with aspirin, a beta-blocker, an angiotensin-converting enzyme inhibitor and a statin. In view of his age it might be worth doing an exercise test to ensure that there is no evidence of ischaemia at a low workload.

Summary ★
Old anterior myocardial infarction.

ME See p. 103

IP See pp. 243 and 250

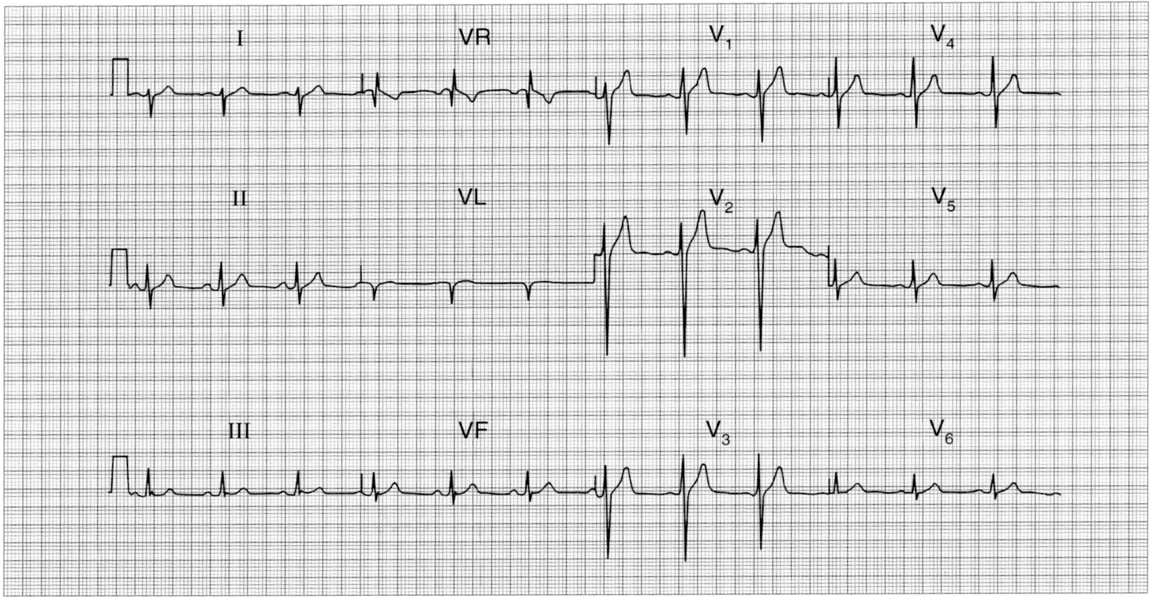

ECG 82 This ECG was recorded from an asymptomatic 30-year-old man at a routine examination. Is it normal?

ANSWER 82

The ECG shows:

- Sinus rhythm
- Right axis deviation (S waves bigger than R waves in lead I, large R waves in lead VR, very small R waves and deep S waves in lead VL)
- Notched QRS complexes in lead III
- Otherwise entirely normal QRS complexes and T waves

Clinical interpretation

Right axis deviation can be a feature of right ventricular hypertrophy, but in tall thin people it is a normal variant. The notched QRS complexes in lead III are normal, though if present in all leads they could be the 'J' waves of hypothermia.

What to do

Examine the patient and exclude right ventricular hypertrophy (you should have done this before recording the ECG!).

Summary ★
Normal ECG.

IP See p. 62

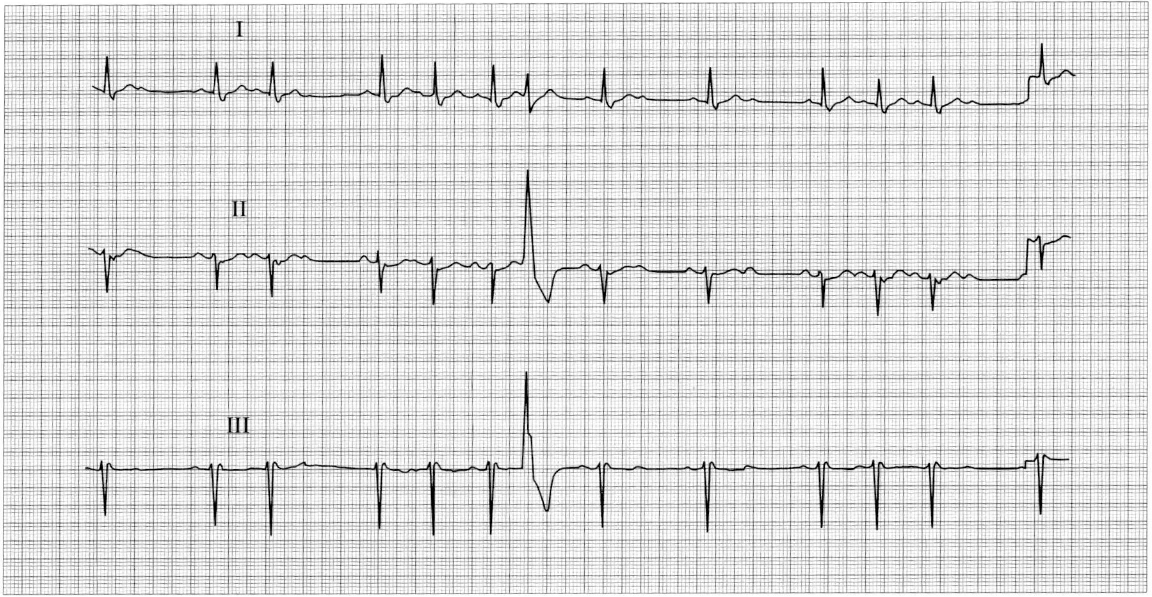

ECG 83 This ECG was recorded from a 70-year-old woman who had complained of attacks of dizziness for about a year. Note that only leads I, II and III are shown, but there are three abnormalities. How should this woman be treated?

ANSWER 83

The ECG shows:

- Variable rhythm
- Sinus rhythm at times
- One ventricular extrasystole
- Intermittent second degree (both Mobitz type 2 and 2:1) heart block
- Left axis deviation

Clinical interpretation

There are two varieties of second degree block here – Mobitz type 2 at the beginning of the record (single non-conducted beats), with 2:1 block for four sinus beats later. The ventricular extrasystole is not significant, but the left axis deviation indicates left anterior hemiblock.

What to do

The full ECG may indicate the underlying disease. It may show, for example, an old anterior myocardial infarction. A 24 h ambulatory ECG tape-recording may reveal the rhythm associated with dizziness. Whatever these findings, however, the patient needs a permanent pacemaker.

Summary ★★
Second degree block with left axis deviation.

ME See pp. 16 and 31

IP See p. 140

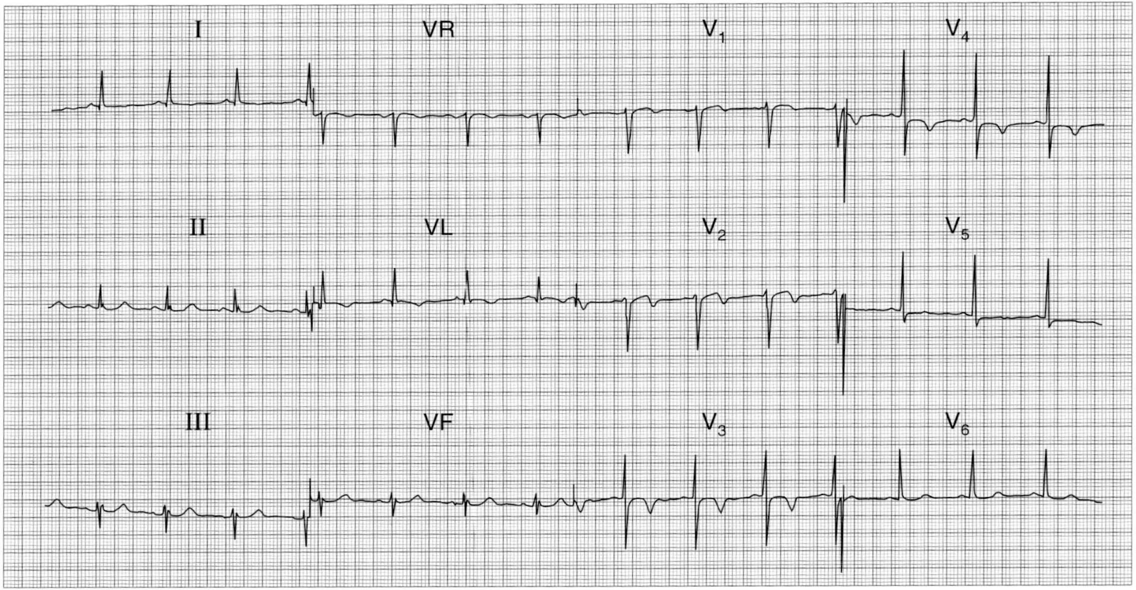

ECG 84 This ECG was recorded in the A & E department from a 60-year-old man who had had intermittent central chest pain for 24 h. What does it show and how should he be managed?

ANSWER 84

The ECG shows:

- Sinus rhythm
- Normal conduction intervals
- Normal axis
- Normal QRS complexes
- Normal ST segments
- T wave inversion in leads I, VL, V_2–V_4

Clinical interpretation

This ECG shows an anterior non-Q wave infarction of uncertain age.

What to do

This patient clearly has an acute coronary syndrome. He must be admitted and treated with low-molecular-weight heparin, a nitrate and a beta-blocker. If the pain does not settle quickly, the use of a glycoprotein IIb/IIIa inhibitor such as tirofiban or abciximab should be considered as a prelude to early angiography and angioplasty.

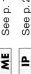

Summary ★
Anterior non-Q wave infarction.

ME See p. 103

IP See p. 266

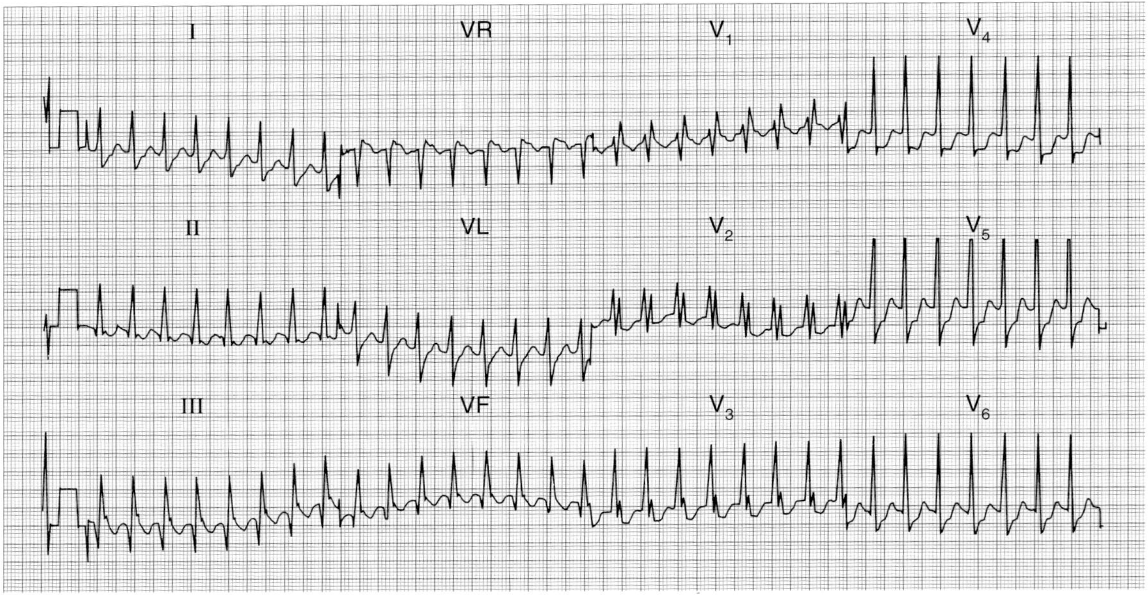

ECG 85 A 25-year-old man, known to have an atrial septal defect, was admitted to hospital as an emergency because of palpitations. His heart rate was 170/min, his blood pressure was 140/80 and there were no signs of heart failure. What is the cardiac rhythm and what would you do?

ANSWER 85

The ECG shows:

- Broad-complex tachycardia, rate 170/min
- No clear P waves but possibly some P waves visible in lead VR
- Normal axis
- Right bundle branch block pattern
- Horizontal ST segment depression in V_4, V_5

Clinical interpretation

The QRS complex duration is 120 ms, the axis is normal, and the QRS complexes show the classic right bundle branch block pattern. It is likely that this is a supraventricular tachycardia with right bundle branch block, and this would be certain if we were sure of the existence of P waves in lead VR. This is either an atrial or a junctional tachycardia. The ST segment depression suggests ischaemia.

What to do

If the patient is known to have an atrial septal defect he is likely to have right bundle branch block, and this could be confirmed in pre-existing hospital records. The initial treatment is carotid sinus massage, and if this proves ineffective, intravenous adenosine.

Summary ★★★

Supraventricular tachycardia (possibly atrial) with right bundle branch block.

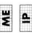

ME See pp. 36 and 74

IP See p. 170

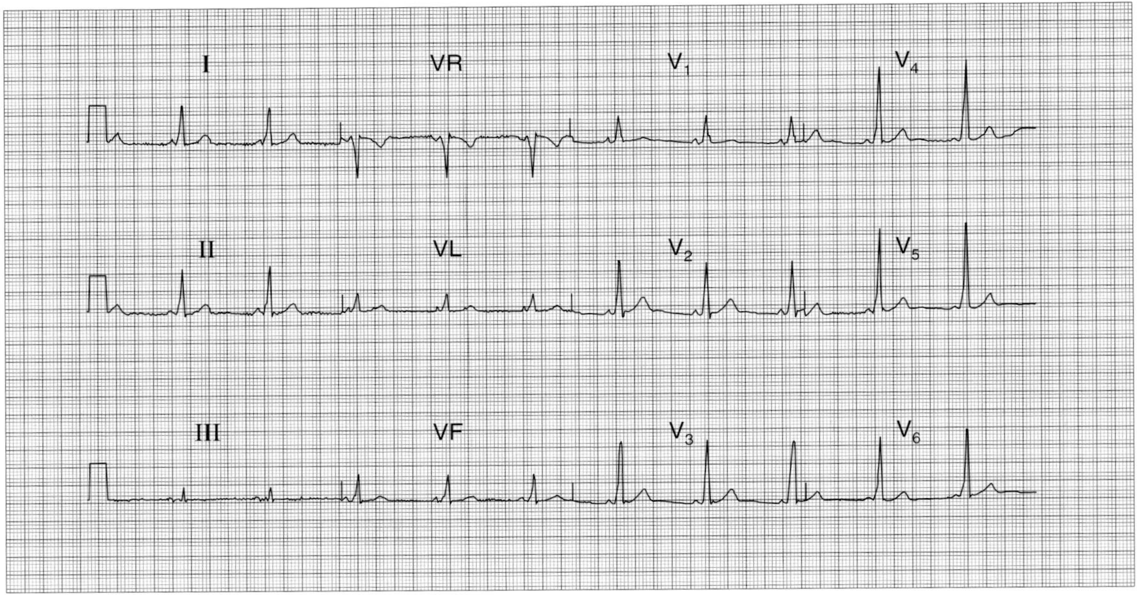

ECG 86 A 30-year-old woman, who had a baby 3 months previously, complains of breathlessness, and this is her ECG. What is the problem?

ANSWER 86

The ECG shows:

- Sinus rhythm
- Short PR interval at 100 ms
- Normal axis
- Normal QRS duration
- Slurred upstroke to QRS (delta wave)
- Dominant R wave in lead V_1
- Normal ST segments and T waves

Clinical interpretation

This ECG shows a Wolff–Parkinson–White syndrome type A, which is characterized by a dominant R wave in lead V_1.

What to do

The catch here is that the dominant R wave in lead V_1 may be mistakenly thought to be due to right ventricular hypertrophy. In a young woman who complains of breathlessness after a pregnancy, pulmonary embolism is obviously a possibility, and this might well cause ECG evidence of right ventricular hypertrophy, but in the presence of a Wolff–Parkinson–White syndrome this would be very difficult to diagnose from the ECG. The only thing that might help would be the appearance of right axis, which is not part of the Wolff–Parkinson–White syndrome, and is not present here.

Summary ★★
Wolff–Parkinson–White syndrome type A.

ME See p. 81

IP See pp. 117 and 120

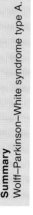

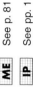

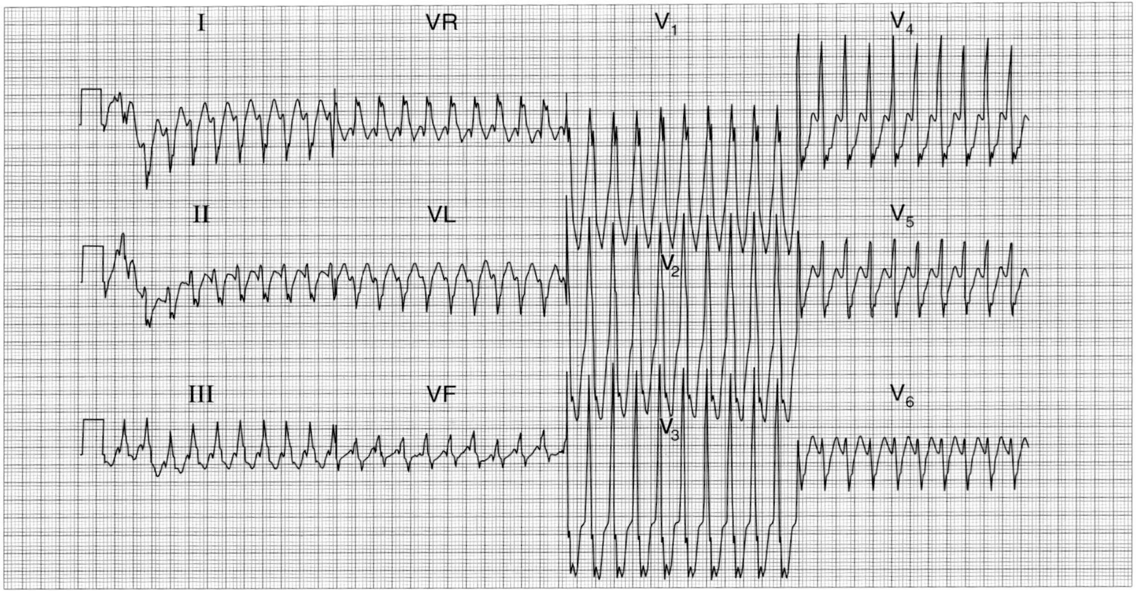

ECG 87 A 30-year-old man, who had had brief episodes of palpitations for at least 10 years, was seen during an attack in the A & E department and this is his ECG. What is the rhythm, and what would you do immediately, and in the long term?

ANSWER 87

The ECG shows:

- Broad complex tachycardia at about 250/min
- No P waves visible
- Right axis
- QRS duration of about 180 ms
- QRS complexes point upwards in lead V_1 and downwards in lead V_6 – no concordance
- Right bundle branch block QRS configuration; the first R wave peak is higher than the second peak

Clinical interpretation

There are essentially three causes of a broad complex tachycardia: ventricular tachycardia, supraventricular tachycardia with bundle branch block, and the Wolff–Parkinson–White syndrome. The key to the diagnosis lies in the ECG when the patient is in sinus rhythm, but this is not always available. Patients with a broad complex tachycardia in the context of an acute myocardial infarction must be assumed to have a ventricular tachycardia, but that does not apply here. In this record the QRS is not very broad, the axis is to the right, and there is no concordance of the QRS complexes – all pointing to a supraventricular origin. In favour of a ventricular tachycardia is the fact that the height of the primary R wave is greater than that of the secondary R wave. Taking these features together with the clinical picture, the rhythm is probably supraventricular.

What to do

Carotid sinus pressure is the first move. If there is severe haemodynamic compromise the patient may need urgent electrical cardioversion, but intravenous flecainide would be a reasonable first choice. In fact the arrhythmia terminated spontaneously, revealing a short PR interval and a QRS complex with a delta wave. So this patient has a Wolff–Parkinson–White syndrome, and needs an electrophysiological study with a view to ablation of the accessory tract.

Summary ★★★
Broad complex tachycardia due to a Wolff–Parkinson–White syndrome.

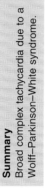

ME See p. 81
IP See p. 127

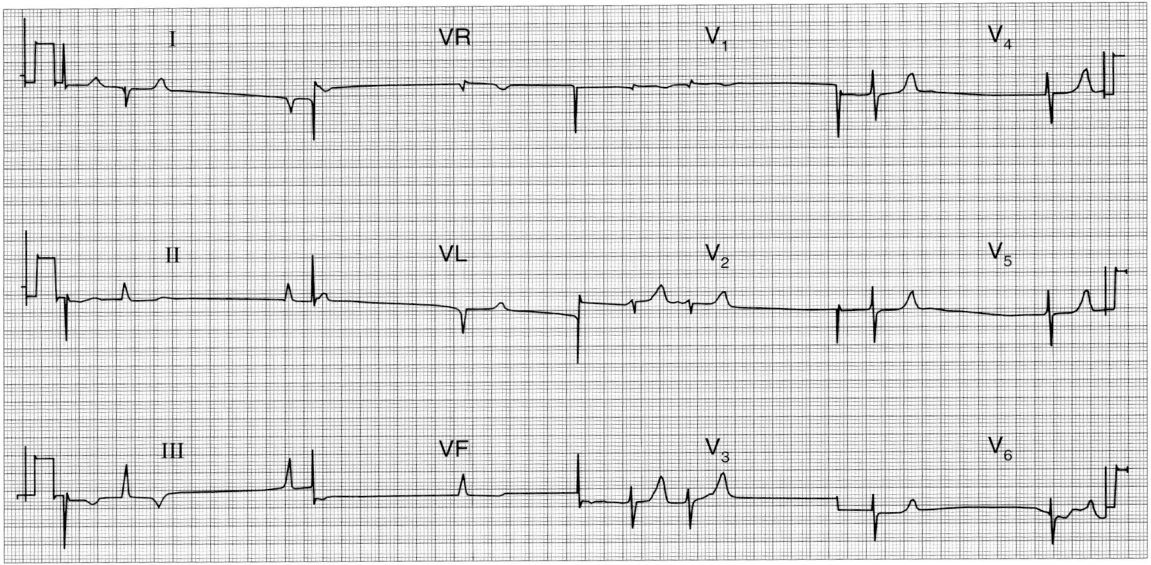

ECG 88 A 65-year-old woman with rheumatic heart disease, who had had severe heart failure for years, was admitted with increasing breathlessness and ankle swelling. Despite having been treated with angiotensin-converting enzyme inhibitors and diuretics, there was evidence of severe heart failure. Having seen the ECG what more do you want to know?

ANSWER 88

The ECG shows:

- Uncertain rhythm – no P waves, irregular QRS but no 'fibrillation' activity
- Right axis
- Normal QRS complexes except for a deep S wave in V_6
- Symmetrically peaked T waves
- Inverted T waves in leads III and VF

Clinical interpretation

The absence of atrial activity and the peaked T waves are consistent with hyperkalaemia. The right axis and deep S waves in lead V_6 could indicate right ventricular hypertrophy and could result from chronic lung disease. The inverted T waves in leads III and VF suggest ischaemia.

What to do

Find out what the patient's medication has been and check the electrolyte levels. This woman had been treated with a combination of captopril 25 mg, three times daily (which tends to raise the serum potassium level) and three co-amilofruse tablets per 24 h (frusemide 40 mg plus amiloride 5 mg in each tablet). The combination of captopril and amiloride causes marked potassium retention, and in this case the serum potassium level was 7.4 mmol/l.

When the hyperkalaemia was corrected, sinus rhythm with clear P waves was restored and the peaked T waves became normal. The right axis, clockwise rotation and inverted T waves in the inferior leads persisted.

Summary ★★★
Hyperkalaemia.

ME See p. 108

IP See p. 366

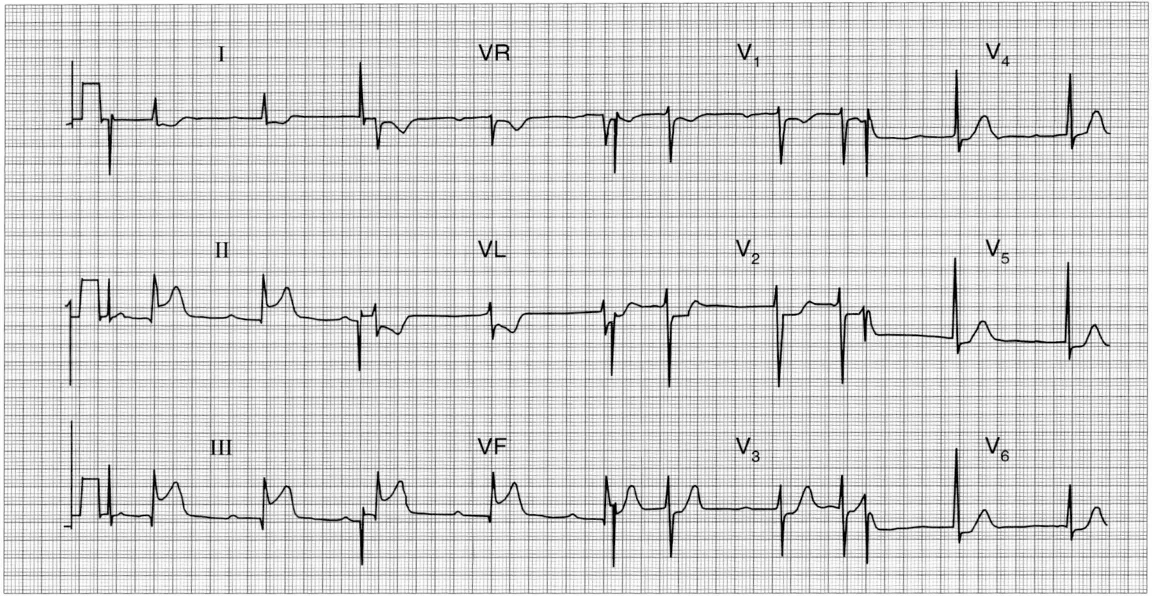

ECG 89 This ECG was recorded from a 55-year-old man who was admitted to hospital as an emergency with severe central chest pain that had been present for about an hour. He was pale, cold and clammy; his blood pressure was 100/80, but there were no signs of heart failure. What does this ECG show? Does anything about it surprise you?

ANSWER 89

The ECG shows:

- Sinus rhythm, rate 55/min
- First degree block (PR interval 350 ms)
- Normal axis
- Small Q waves in leads II, III, VF
- Raised ST segments in leads II, III, VF
- Depressed ST segments and inverted T waves in leads I, VL
- Slight ST segment depression in the chest leads

Clinical interpretation

Acute inferior myocardial infarction with anterolateral ischaemia, and first degree block. Patients who are in pain with an acute myocardial infarction usually have a sinus tachycardia, but here vagal overactivity is causing a bradycardia.

What to do

First degree block is not important in itself, but with evidence of vagal overactivity, atropine should be given. Otherwise this patient can be treated in the usual way with pain relief, aspirin, and thrombolytics.

Summary ★
Acute inferior myocardial infarction with first degree block.

ME See p. 96
IP See p. 238

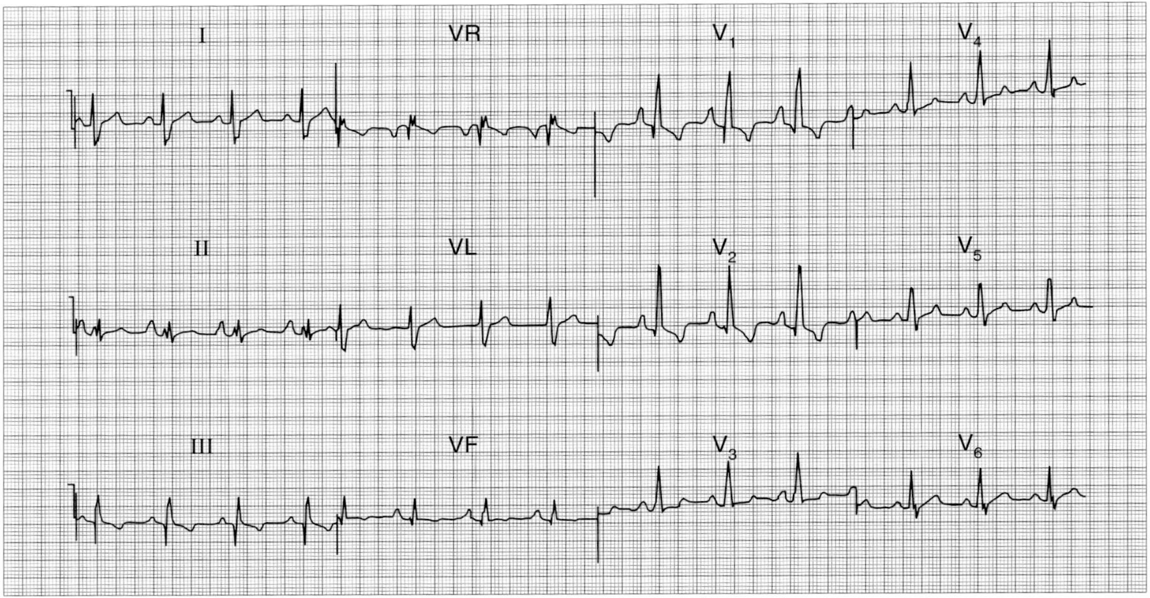

ECG 90 This ECG was recorded from a 17-year-old girl who was breathless, had marked ankle swelling with signs of right heart failure, and who had been known to have a heart murmur since birth. She was acyanotic. What ECG abnormalities can you identify and can you suggest a diagnosis?

ANSWER 90

The ECG shows:

- Sinus rhythm
- Markedly peaked P waves (best seen in leads II, V_1)
- Normal axis
- Dominant R wave in lead V_1

Clinical interpretation
The ECG shows right atrial and right ventricular hypertrophy.

What to do
Right atrial hypertrophy is seen with pulmonary hypertension of any cause, tricuspid stenosis, and Ebstein's anomaly. Right ventricular hypertrophy is seen with pulmonary stenosis and pulmonary hypertension. These conditions can all be diagnosed by echocardiography. This patient had Ebstein's anomaly and an atrial septal defect.

Summary ★★
Right atrial and right ventricular hypertrophy.

ME See p. 91
IP See p. 344

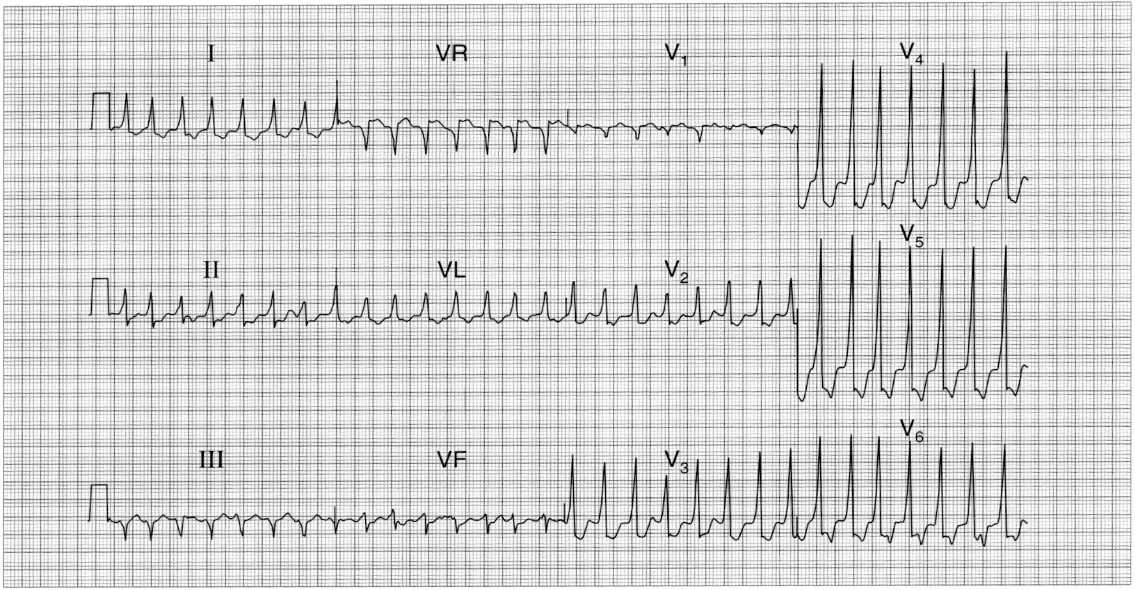

ECG 91 A 35-year-old woman, who had had attacks of what sound like a paroxysmal tachycardia for many years, was seen in the A & E department, and this ECG was recorded. What is the diagnosis?

ANSWER 91

The ECG shows:

- Narrow complex tachycardia at about 170/min
- No P waves visible
- Normal axis
- QRS duration 112 ms
- Slurred upstroke to QRS complexes, best seen in leads V_3–V_4
- Depressed ST segments in leads V_3–V_6
- Inverted T waves in the lateral leads

Clinical interpretation

This is a narrow complex tachycardia, so it is supraventricular. The slurred upstroke to the QRS complex suggests a Wolff–Parkinson–White syndrome, so this is a re-entry tachycardia with depolarization spreading down the accessory pathway. This diagnosis is consistent with the patient's history.

What to do

Carotid sinus pressure is always the first thing to try in patients with a supraventricular tachycardia. In most such patients adenosine is the first drug to use, but in Wolff–Parkinson–White syndromes it must be used with caution. It can block the atrioventricular node and increase conduction through the accessory pathway, and if atrial fibrillation is present this can lead to ventricular fibrillation. Digoxin, verapamil and lignocaine can have the same effect. The safe drugs in this situation are the beta-blockers, flecainide and amiodarone.

Summary ★★

Supraventricular tachycardia and a Wolff–Parkinson–White syndrome.

ME See pp. 74 and 81

IP See pp. 122 and 198

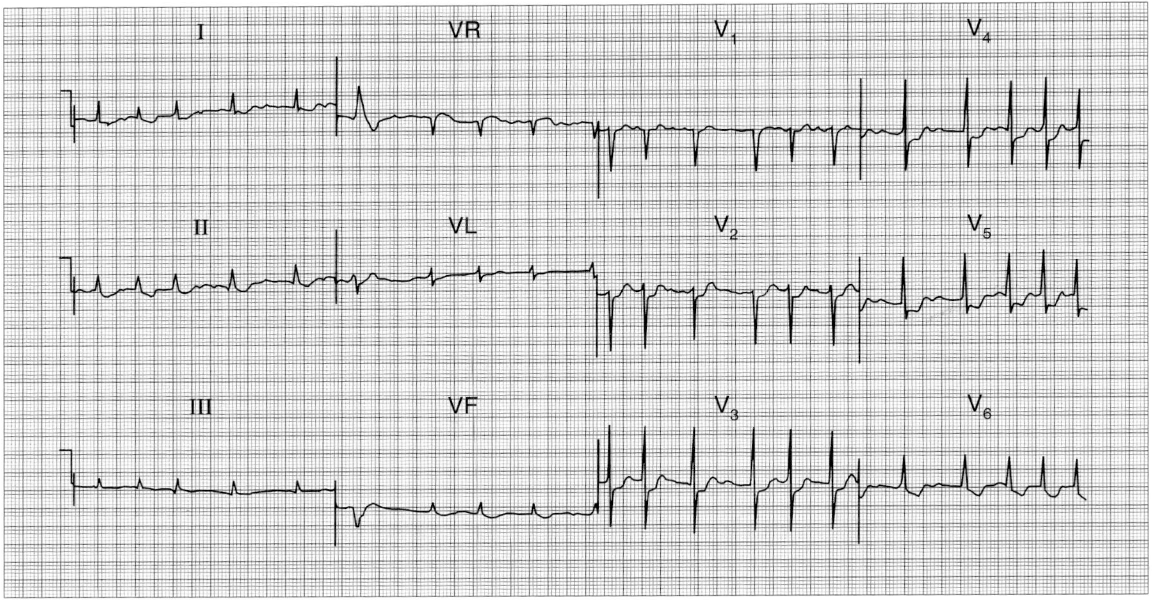

ECG 92 A 60-year-old woman, who has been treated for some time for heart failure, complains of increasing palpitations and weight loss. Having seen this ECG, what diagnoses would you consider, and what would you do?

ANSWER 92

The ECG shows:

- Atrial fibrillation with one ventricular extrasystole
- Ventricular rate 75–150/min
- Normal axis
- Normal QRS complexes
- Horizontal ST segment depression in lead V_4; downward-sloping ST segment depression in lead V_6

Clinical interpretation

The ventricular rate is inadequately controlled (probably explaining the palpitations), although the ST segment in lead V_6 suggests that the patient is being treated with digoxin. The horizontal ST segment depression in lead V_4 suggests ischaemia.

What to do

When a patient has atrial fibrillation but the ventricular rate does not respond to digoxin, think about thyrotoxicosis. This would explain the weight loss, but there are other conditions in which atrial fibrillation and weight loss coexist, including valve disease with infective endocarditis, malignancy with pericardial or cardiac metastases, and alcoholism. Echocardiography, a chest X-ray examination, and measurements of thyroid and liver function tests are needed.

Summary ★★
Atrial fibrillation, with a rapid ventricular rate and evidence of both ischaemia and digoxin effect.

ME See pp. 78 and 100

IP See pp. 267 and 373

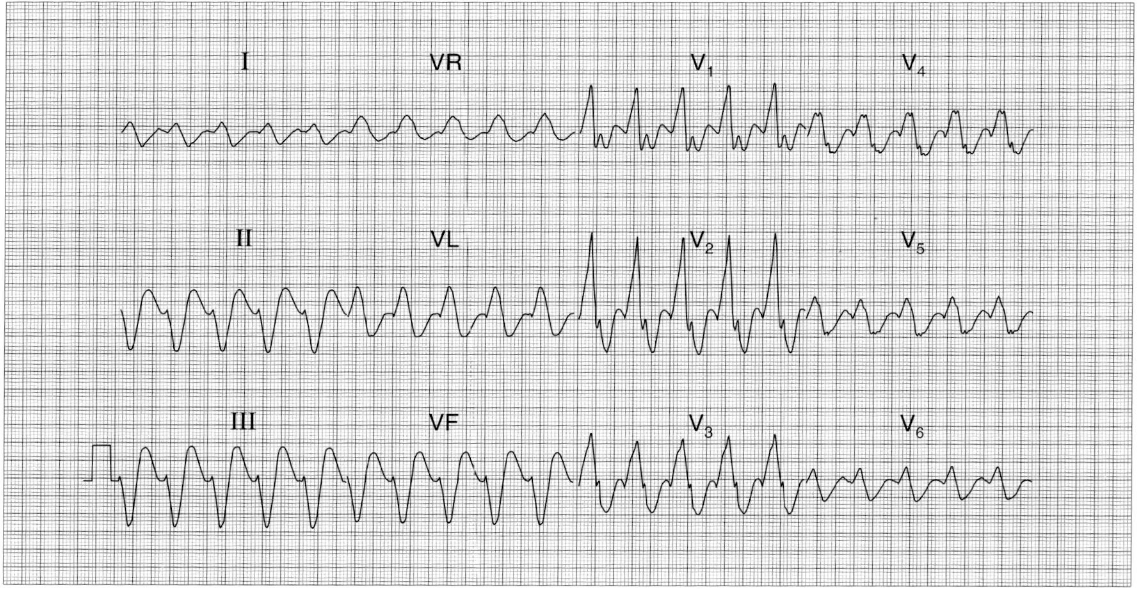

ECG 93 A 60-year-old man, who had been well apart from mild breathlessness on exertion, was admitted to hospital with the sudden onset of pulmonary oedema, and this is his ECG. He had no pain. What is the rhythm, and how will you treat him?

ANSWER 93

The ECG shows:

- Broad complex rhythm at 130/min
- No P waves
- Left axis
- QRS duration 200 ms
- QRS complexes show right bundle branch block configuration
- QRS complexes in the anterior leads are not concordant

Clinical interpretation

The very broad QRS complexes and left axis suggest that this is a ventricular tachycardia. However, the lack of concordance (i.e. the QRS complexes in leads V_1–V_4 are upright, while those in leads V_5–V_6 are predominantly downward) and the right bundle branch block pattern with the secondary R wave peak being higher than the primary peak suggest that this could be a supraventricular rhythm with bundle branch block. Comparison with the patient's ECG when in sinus rhythm is the only way of being certain what the rhythm is.

What to do

If the patient has pulmonary oedema, preparations for DC cardioversion should be made immediately, and while waiting for this he should be treated with diamorphine, intravenous diuretics and lignocaine or intravenous amiodarone. The ECG following cardioversion is shown in the next example.

Summary ★★

Broad complex tachycardia of uncertain aetiology.

ME See p. 75

IP See p. 171

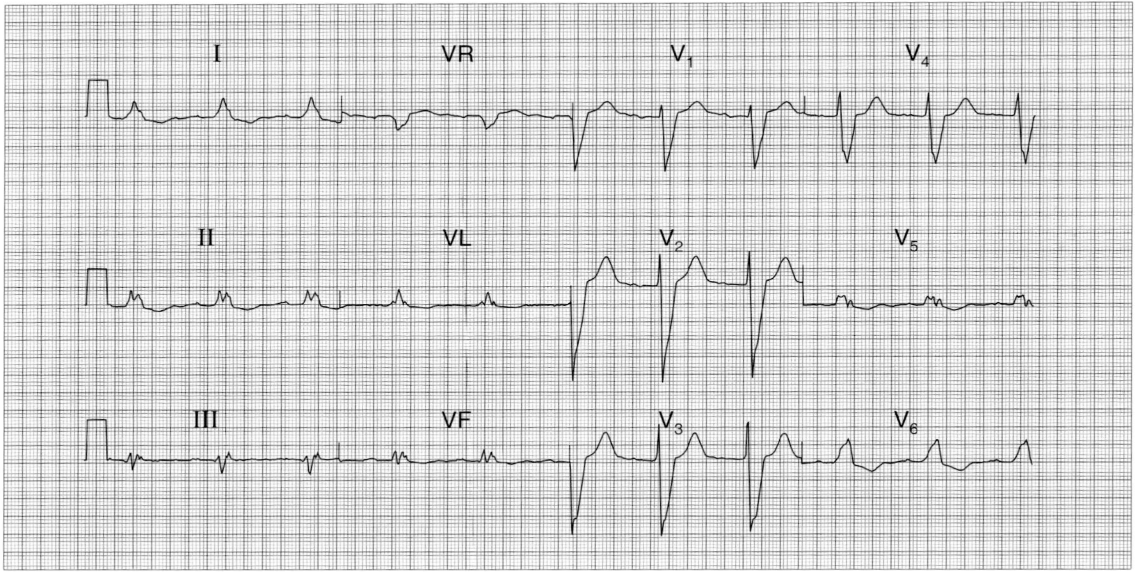

ECG 94 This is another ECG from the 60-year-old man who was admitted with a broad complex tachycardia (see the previous example). This ECG was recorded after cardioversion, when he was well. His troponin level remained normal following admission so he had not had a myocardial infarction. How would you report on this ECG, and what do you think the underlying disease is?

ANSWER 94

The ECG shows:

- Sinus rhythm
- First degree block (PR interval 220 ms)
- Normal axis
- Broad QRS complexes (200 ms)
- Left bundle branch block

Clinical interpretation

Comparison with this patient's previous ECG (see p. 185) shows that when he had the tachycardia there was a change in axis and in QRS configuration. The broad complex tachycardia was therefore almost certainly ventricular in origin. He now has evidence of conduction tissue disease, with first degree block and left bundle branch block. Since chest pain has not been a feature of his illness it seems likely that he has a dilated cardiomyopathy.

What to do

If after treatment with an angiotensin-converting enzyme inhibitor and amiodarone the patient has another episode of ventricular tachycardia, an implanted defibrillator may be needed.

Summary ★★
First degree block and left bundle branch block.

ME See pp. 30 and 39

IP See p. 114

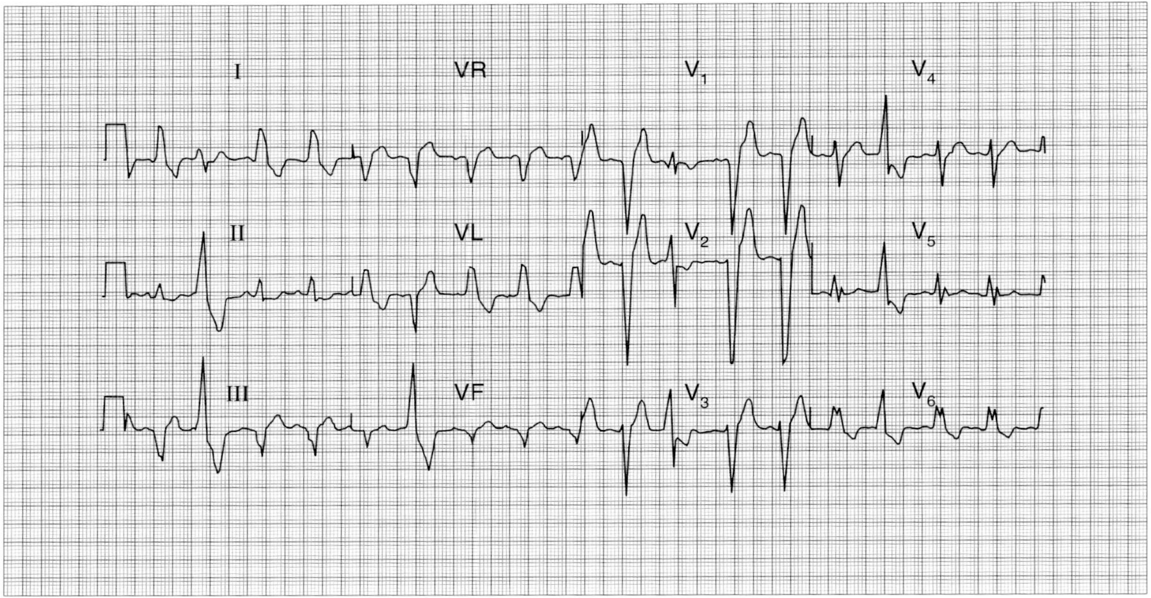

ECG 95 This ECG was recorded from a 50-year-old man admitted to hospital following 2 h of central chest pain that was characteristic of a myocardial infarction. Six months previously, his ECG had been normal. What does this record show and what would you do?

ANSWER 95

The ECG shows:

- Sinus rhythm
- Normal axis
- Ventricular extrasystoles
- Left bundle branch block in the sinus beats

Clinical interpretation

The ventricular extrasystoles can be identified because they have a different morphology from the left bundle branch block pattern, and because they have no preceding P waves. Left bundle branch block masks any changes there might be as the result of a myocardial infarction.

What to do

The left bundle branch block has evidently developed in the last 6 months, and the history suggests a myocardial infarction. Provided there are no contraindications, a thrombolytic agent should be given. The ventricular extrasystoles should not be treated.

Summary ★★★

Sinus rhythm with left bundle branch block and ventricular extrasystoles.

ME See pp. 39 and 64

IP See p. 259

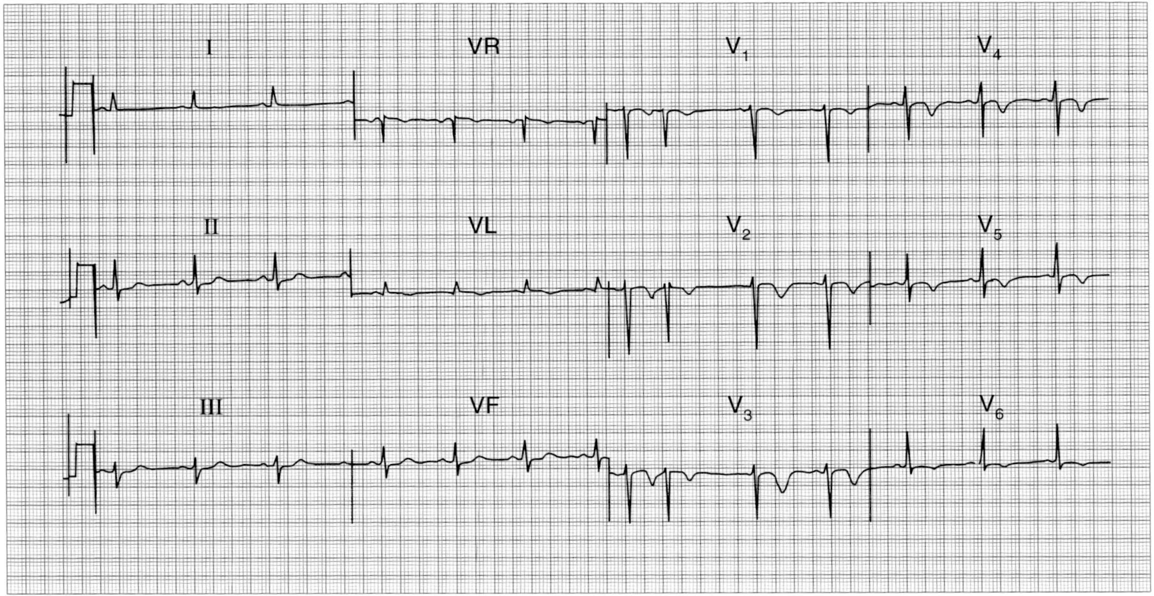

ECG 96 A 50-year-old man was admitted to hospital as an emergency, having had central chest pain for 1 h. By the time he was seen in the A & E department he was pain-free and there were no abnormalities on examination. This is his ECG. What does it show, and what would you do?

ANSWER 96

The ECG shows:

- Sinus rhythm with one supraventricular extrasystole (there appears to be an abnormal P wave in lead V_1, so this is atrial in origin)
- Normal axis
- Normal QRS complexes
- Inverted T waves in leads VL, V_1–V_6

Clinical interpretation

There are many causes of inverted T waves, and ECGs should always be interpreted as part of the overall clinical picture. In this case the history suggests a myocardial infarction, and the ECG is characteristic of an acute anterior non-Q wave infarction.

What to do

The *immediate* risk is low and there is no evidence for benefit from thrombolysis. Although the patient is now asymptomatic he should remain in hospital for observation. The risk of reinfarction in the next 3 months is relatively high compared with the risk following a Q wave infarction, and further investigation is needed.

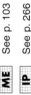

Summary ★
Anterolateral non-Q wave myocardial infarction.

ME See p. 103

IP See p. 266

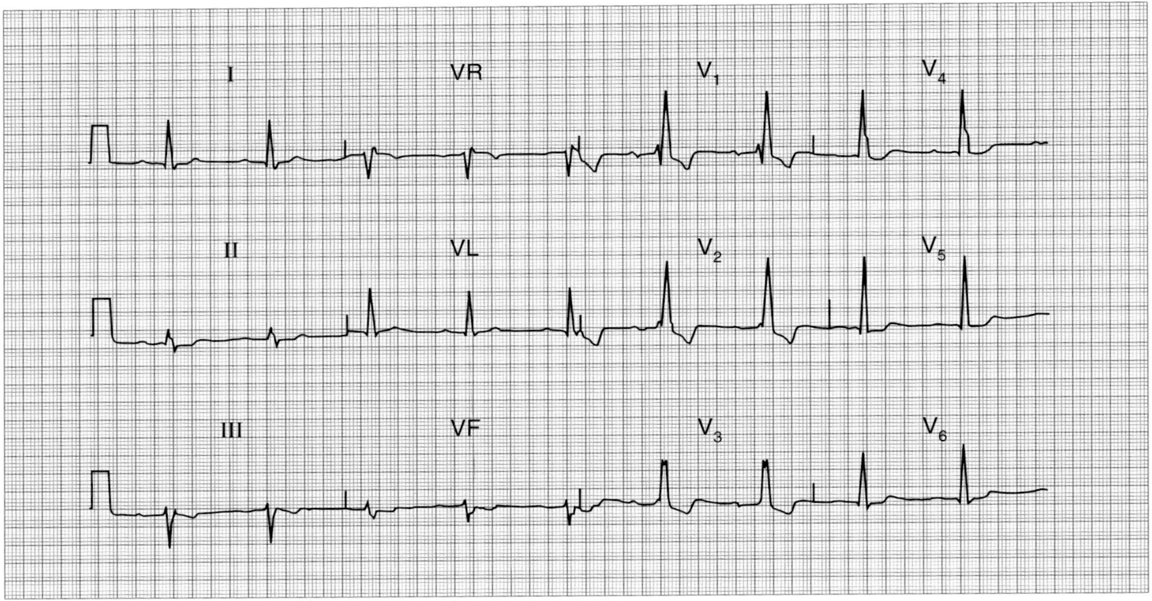

ECG 97 This ECG was recorded as part of the routine preoperative assessment of a 65-year-old man who had no cardiovascular symptoms, and whose heart was clinically normal. What does it show? Is any action necessary?

ANSWER 97

The ECG shows:

- Sinus rhythm
- First degree block (PR interval 280 ms)
- Normal axis
- Right bundle branch block

Clinical interpretation
The first degree block indicates conduction delay in the His bundle or left bundle branch, in addition to complete block of the right bundle branch.

What to do
The danger is that complete heart block will develop, though the present situation could remain stable for a prolonged period. There is certainly no urgency regarding treatment, but many cardiologists would recommend the insertion of a permanent pacemaker. No other treatment would be helpful. Consider the possibility that he has an anterior septal defect.

Summary ★
Sinus rhythm, first degree block and right bundle branch block.

ME See pp. 30 and 37

IP See p. 137

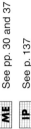

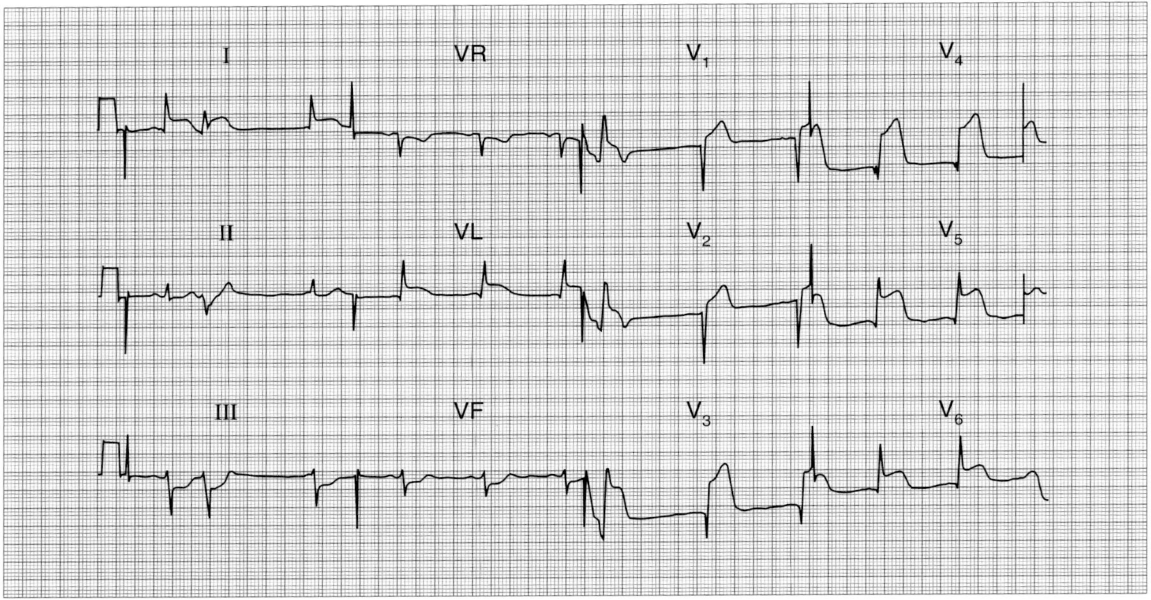

ECG 98 This ECG was recorded from a 50-year-old man who had had severe chest pain for 1 h. What does it show and what would you do?

ANSWER 98

The ECG shows:

- Sinus rhythm with ventricular extrasystoles
- Normal axis
- Q waves in leads V_3–V_5
- Raised ST segments in leads I, VL, V_3–V_6
- Depressed ST segments in leads III, VF

Clinical interpretation

Ventricular extrasystoles associated with an acute anterolateral myocardial infarction.

What to do

The patient should be given diamorphine and aspirin immediately, and thrombolysis as soon as possible. The extrasystoles should not be treated.

Summary ★

Acute anterolateral myocardial infarction with ventricular extrasystoles.

ME See p. 98

IP See p. 242

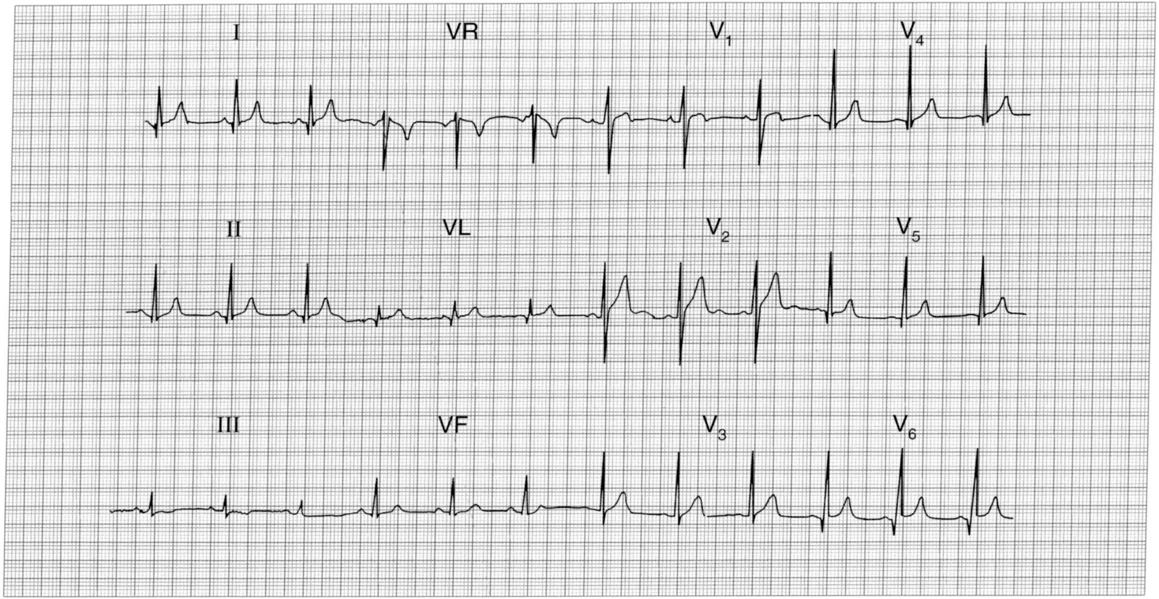

ECG 99 This ECG was recorded from a 30-year-old man who complained of chest pain: the pain did not appear to be cardiac in origin, and physical examination was normal. Can this man be allowed to hold a commercial driving licence?

ANSWER 99

The ECG shows:

- Sinus rhythm
- Normal axis
- Small Q waves, especially prominent in leads I, II, V_4–V_6
- Otherwise normal QRS complexes
- T wave inversion in lead III but not VF

Clinical interpretation

These Q waves are quite deep but only 40 ms in duration, and they are most prominent in the lateral leads. They represent septal depolarization, not an old lateral infarction. An inverted T wave in lead III but not in lead VF is a normal variant.

What to do

The ECG is normal, and if the man has no other evidence of heart disease he can hold a commercial driving licence. If in doubt an exercise test should be performed.

Summary ★★
Normal ECG.

IP See p. 89

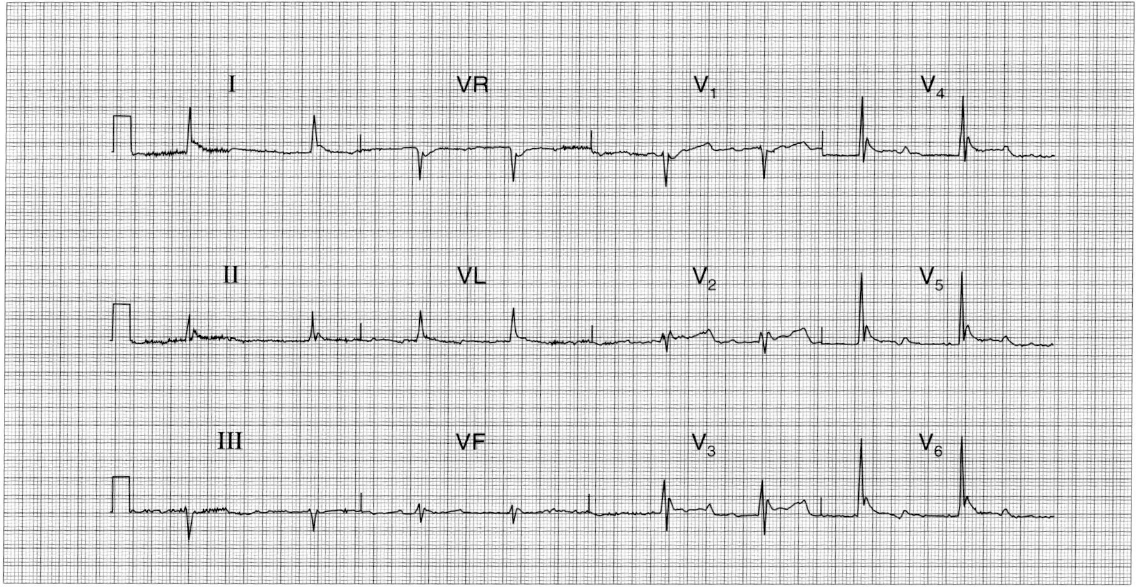

ECG 100 This ECG was recorded from an 80-year-old woman who had been found unconscious with physical signs suggesting a stroke. Any comments?

ANSWER 100

The ECG shows:

- Atrial fibrillation with a ventricular rate of 50/min
- QRS duration prolonged at 160 ms
- Prominent 'J' waves, best seen in leads V_3–V_6
- Widespread but non-specific ST/T changes

Clinical interpretation

The atrial fibrillation may or may not be related to her stroke – she may have had a cerebral embolus, or she may have both coronary and cerebrovascular disease. The slow ventricular rate and the 'J' waves indicate hypothermia, and her core temperature was 25°C. ECGs from hypothermic patients seldom show 'J' waves as clearly as this because there are too many artefacts due to shivering – but this patient was too cold to shiver. She did not survive.

Summary ★★★
Atrial fibrillation and hypothermia.

IP See p. 358

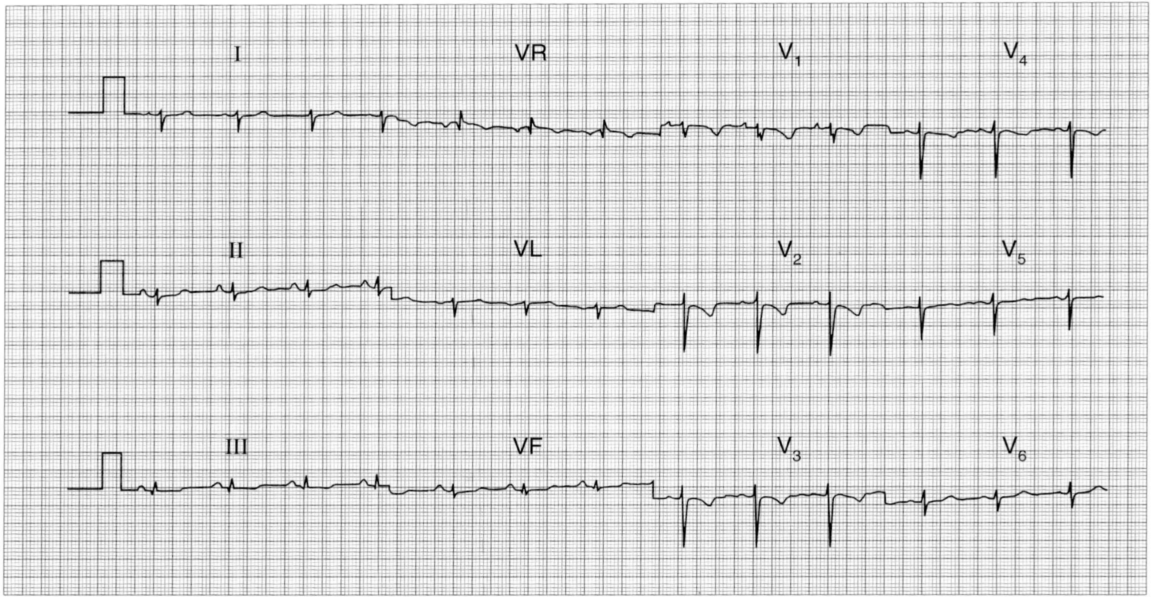

ECG 101 A 32-year-old woman, who had a normal pregnancy and delivery 3 months previously, was seen in the out-patient department complaining of breathlessness and dizziness on exertion. She had had no chest pain. Does her ECG help with her diagnosis and treatment?

ANSWER 101

The ECG shows:

- Sinus rhythm
- Right axis deviation
- Normal QRS complexes except for an RSR pattern in lead V_1 and deep S waves in lead V_6
- Inverted T waves in leads V_1–V_4

Clinical interpretation

The right axis deviation, the deep S waves in lead V_6 ('clockwise rotation') and the inverted T waves in the chest leads are all characteristic of marked right ventricular hypertrophy: the only missing feature is the absence of dominant R waves in lead V_1. Note how the T wave inversion is at a maximum in lead V_1 and becomes progressively less marked from lead V_2 to V_4.

What to do

In the context of a delivery 3 months previously, this ECG pattern of right ventricular hypertrophy almost certainly indicates multiple small pulmonary emboli causing pulmonary hypertension. A lung scan would confirm this diagnosis and anticoagulants are needed urgently.

Summary ★★
Right ventricular hypertrophy.

ME See pp. 91 and 117

IP See p. 289

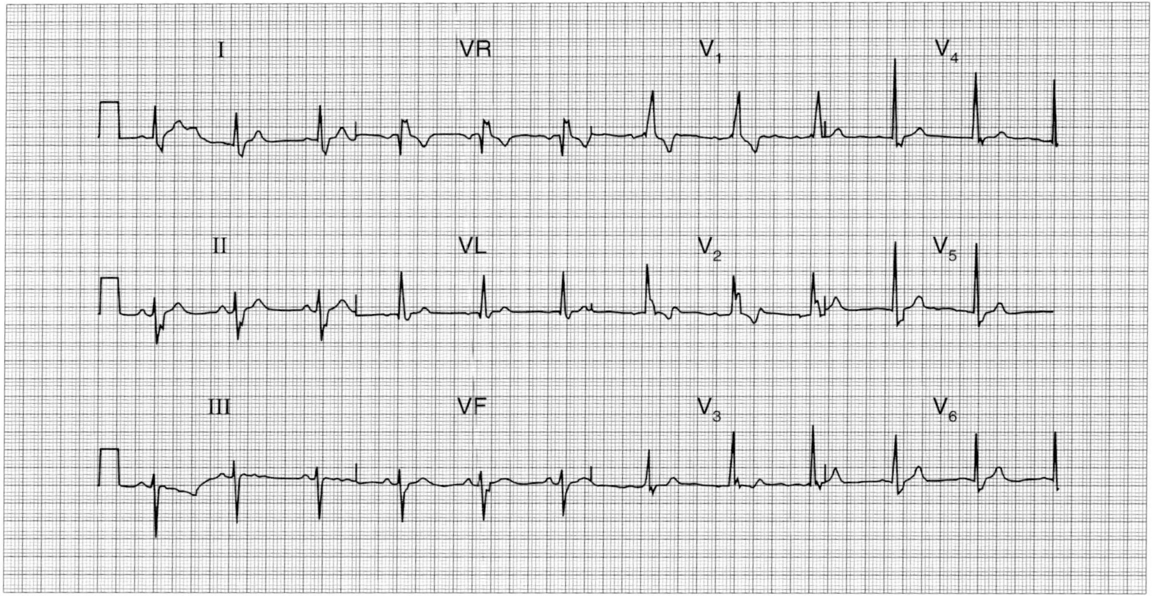

ECG 102 This ECG was recorded from a fit 60-year-old man at a routine medical examination. What does it show and what would you recommend?

ANSWER 102

The ECG shows:

- Sinus rhythm
- Normal PR interval
- Left axis deviation
- Right bundle branch block

Clinical interpretation

The combination of left axis deviation (also called left anterior hemiblock, because it is due to block of the anterior fascicle of the left bundle branch) and right bundle branch block is called bifascicular block. Atrioventricular conduction depends on the posterior fascicle of the left bundle branch.

What to do

Progression to complete block can occur but is relatively rare. In the absence of symptoms, standard UK practice would be *not* to insert a permanent pacemaker.

Summary ★★

Left axis deviation and right bundle branch block – bifascicular block.

ME See p. 48

IP See pp. 140 and 146

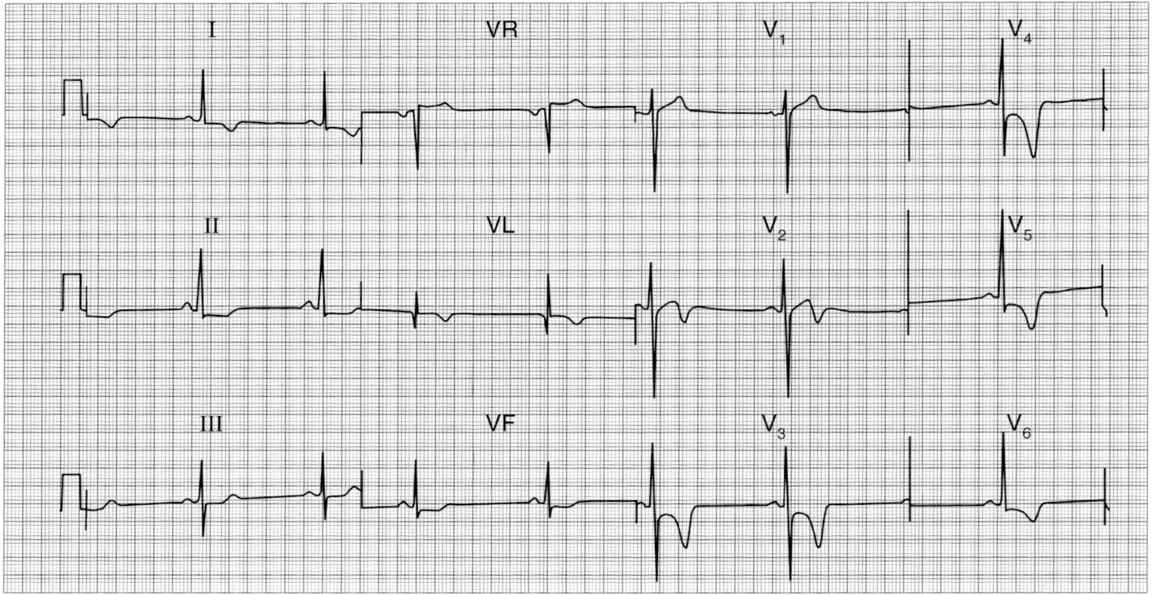

ECG 103 This ECG was recorded as part of a routine examination of a healthy 25-year-old professional athlete. There were no abnormal physical findings. What does it show and what would you do?

ANSWER 103

The ECG shows:

- Sinus rhythm
- Normal axis
- Normal QRS complexes apart from narrow Q waves in lead VL
- Marked T wave inversion in leads I, VL, V_2–V_6

Clinical interpretation

If this ECG had been recorded from a middle-aged man presenting with acute chest pain, the diagnosis would be an anterior non-Q wave infarction, or possibly an early lateral Q wave infarction. The ECGs of athletes can show ST segment and T wave changes due to left ventricular hypertrophy, but anteroseptal T wave inversion of this degree in a healthy young man almost certainly represents hypertrophic cardiomyopathy.

What to do

Echocardiography will confirm the diagnosis. Ambulatory ECG tape-recording will show whether the patient is having ventricular arrhythmias. He must not play competitive sports and his close relatives should be screened.

Summary ★★★
Probable hypertrophic cardiomyopathy.

IP See p. 117 and 120

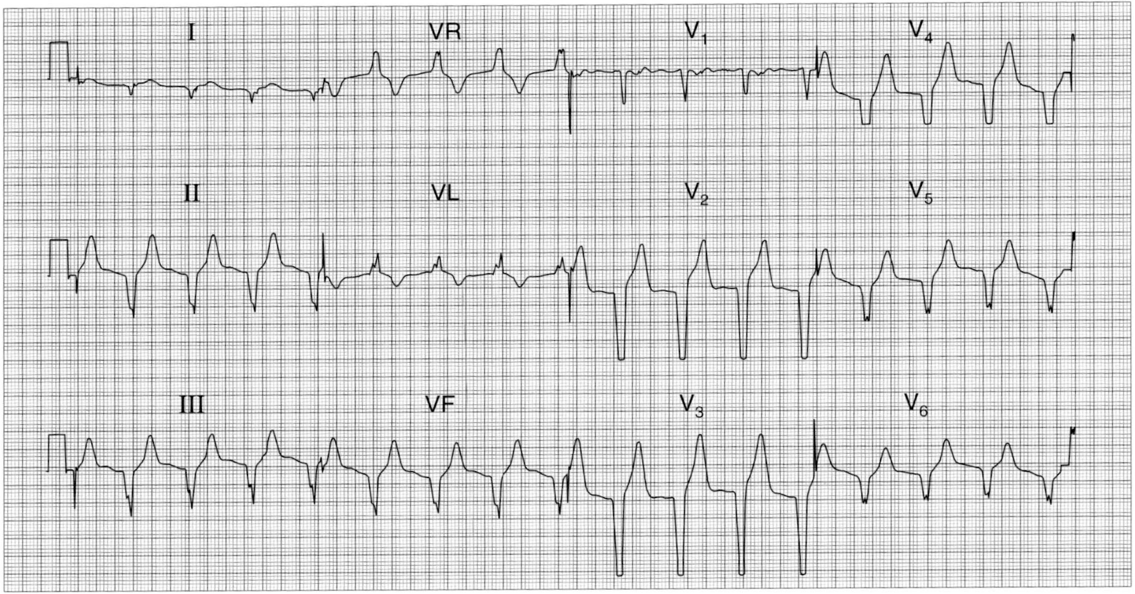

ECG 104 This ECG was recorded from a 45-year-old man, who had been admitted to a coronary care unit with a myocardial infarction and who was recovering well. What is the rhythm, and what would you do?

ANSWER 104

The ECG shows:

- Broad complex rhythm at 90/min
- No P waves
- Marked left axis
- QRS duration 160 ms
- All chest leads show a downward QRS complex (concordance)

Clinical interpretation
If the heart rate were fast there would be little difficulty in recognizing this as ventricular tachycardia, and this rhythm used to be called 'slow VT'. It is, however, an accelerated idioventricular rhythm.

What to do
This rhythm is quite commonly seen in patients with an acute myocardial infarction, and indeed is not uncommon in ambulatory ECG records from normal people. It never causes problems, and it is important not to attempt to treat it: suppressing any 'escape' rhythm may lead to a dangerous bradycardia.

Summary ★★★
Accelerated idioventricular rhythm.

ME See p. 63

IP See pp. 35 and 36

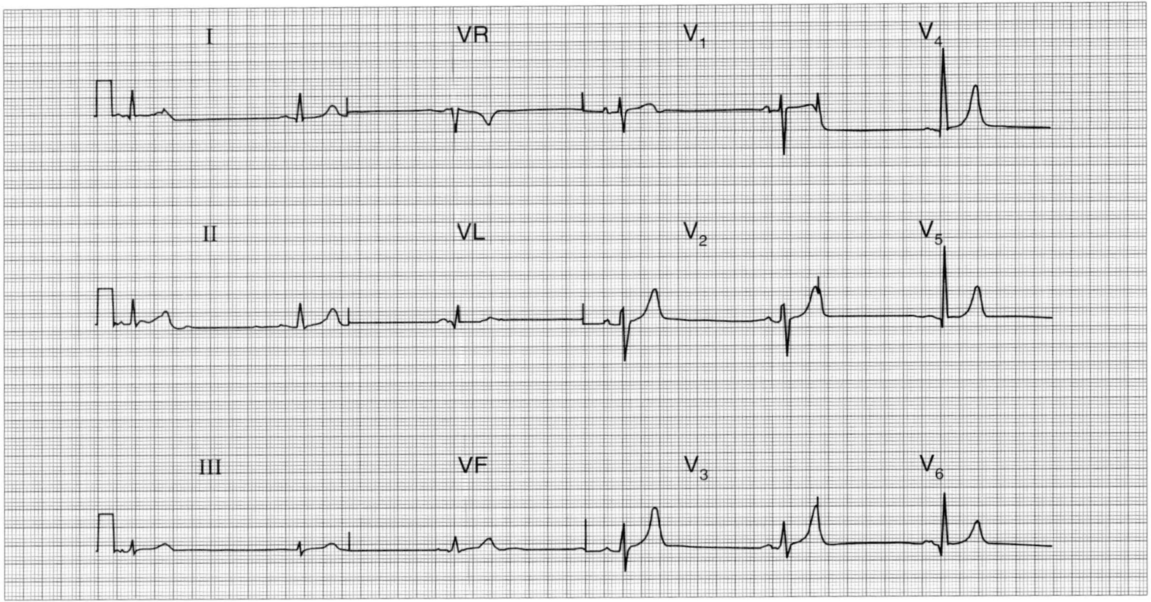

ECG 105 This ECG was recorded from a 50-year-old man who had hypertension but was otherwise well. Despite showing four possible 'abnormalities', is the trace actually normal?

ANSWER 105

The ECG shows:

- Sinus rhythm, rate 34/min
- Normal axis
- Bifid P waves, best seen in the lateral leads
- Small narrow Q waves in the lateral leads
- Normal QRS complexes
- Peaked T waves

Clinical interpretation

Sinus bradycardia can be due to physical fitness, vagal overactivity or myxoedema. In a hypertensive patient, beta-blocker treatment is the likely explanation. The bifid P waves may indicate left atrial hypertrophy ('P mitrale'), but can be normal. The lateral Q waves are normal, representing septal depolarization. The peaked T waves could be due to hyperkalaemia but are more often a normal variant.

What to do

Check the serum potassium level.

Summary ★★
Normal ECG.

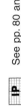

IP See pp. 80 and 96

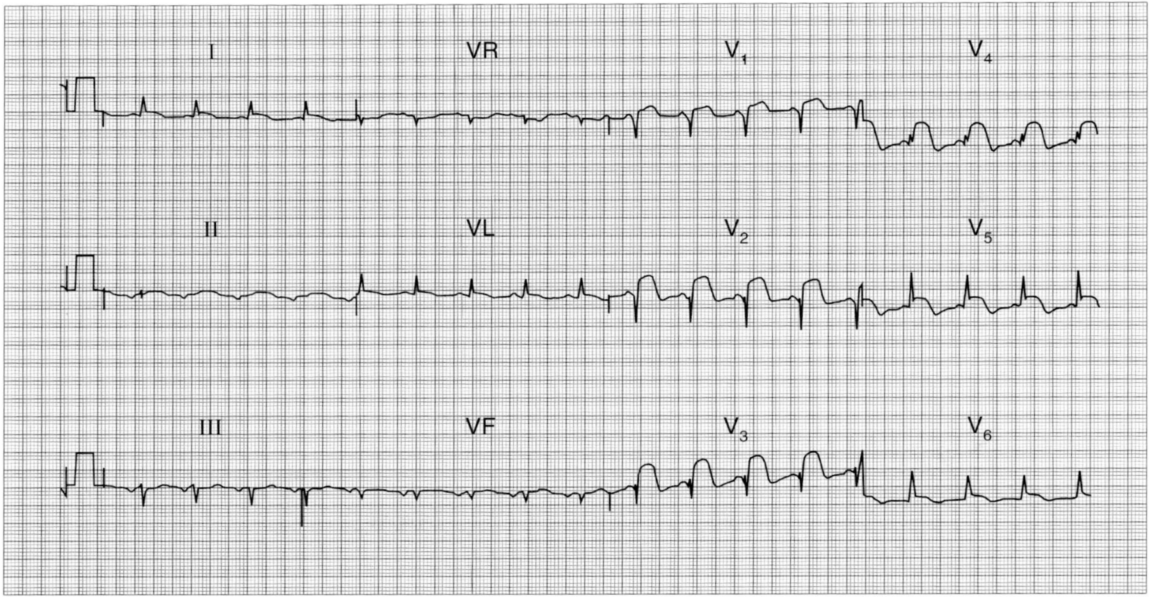

ECG 106 A 48-year-old man is seen in the A & E department with a history of severe chest pain which began 24 h previously, but has now cleared. He is now breathless. What does this ECG show and what treatment is needed?

ANSWER 106

The ECG shows:

- Sinus rhythm
- Normal axis
- Normal QRS complexes
- Raised ST segments in leads I, VL, V_2–V_6

Clinical interpretation

The ECG has the classic appearance of an acute anterolateral myocardial infarction.

What to do

Since this patient's chest pain began more than 24 h ago, thrombolysis is not indicated. The breathlessness suggests that he may have developed left ventricular failure, and he must be admitted to hospital and treated with diuretics and if necessary intravenous nitrates to induce vasodilation. The patient will need long-term treatment with an angiotensin-converting enzyme inhibitor: the best time to begin treatment is a matter for debate but it should be within 2 or 3 days. He will also need long-term treatment with aspirin as a prophylactic against further infarction.

Summary ★
Acute anterolateral myocardial infarction.

ME See p. 98

IP See pp. 242 and 244

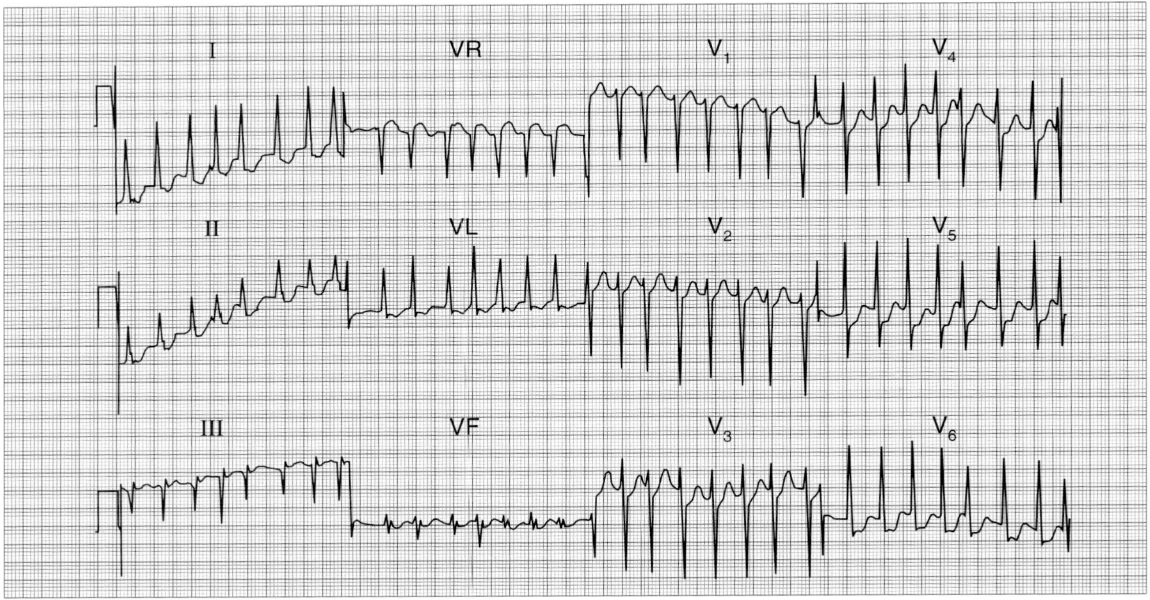

ECG 107 A 50-year-old woman came to the A & E department because of the sudden onset of palpitations and severe breathlessness. What abnormality does this ECG show, and what conditions might be responsible?

ANSWER 107

The ECG shows:

- Atrial fibrillation
- Irregular QRS complexes with a ventricular rate of up to 200/min
- Normal axis
- Height of R waves in lead V_6 plus depth of S waves in lead V_2 is greater than 35 mm, suggesting left ventricular hypertrophy
- Otherwise normal QRS complexes, apart from an RSR pattern in lead VF
- ST segments depressed in leads V_4–V_6, suggesting ischaemia
- Normal T waves

Clinical interpretation

Atrial fibrillation with an uncontrolled ventricular rate. The ischaemic changes in leads V_4 and V_5 are probably related to the heart rate.

What to do

Ischaemia may have been the cause of the atrial fibrillation, or the rapid ventricular rate itself may be responsible for the ischaemic changes. Ischaemia is not a likely primary diagnosis in a 50-year-old woman, and the things to think about are rheumatic heart disease (particularly with mitral stenosis), thyrotoxicosis, alcoholism, and other forms of cardiomyopathy. Immediate treatment of heart failure with diuretics and intravenous nitrates may be necessary, but the ventricular rate is best controlled by digoxin, which can be given intravenously if necessary. DC cardioversion may be necessary if the patient is in severe heart failure, but it is best to establish the underlying cause of the atrial fibrillation first if possible. Remember that a patient with atrial fibrillation probably needs long-term anticoagulants.

Summary ★★

Atrial fibrillation with a rapid ventricular rate and ischaemic changes.

ME See pp. 78 and 102

IP See p. 315

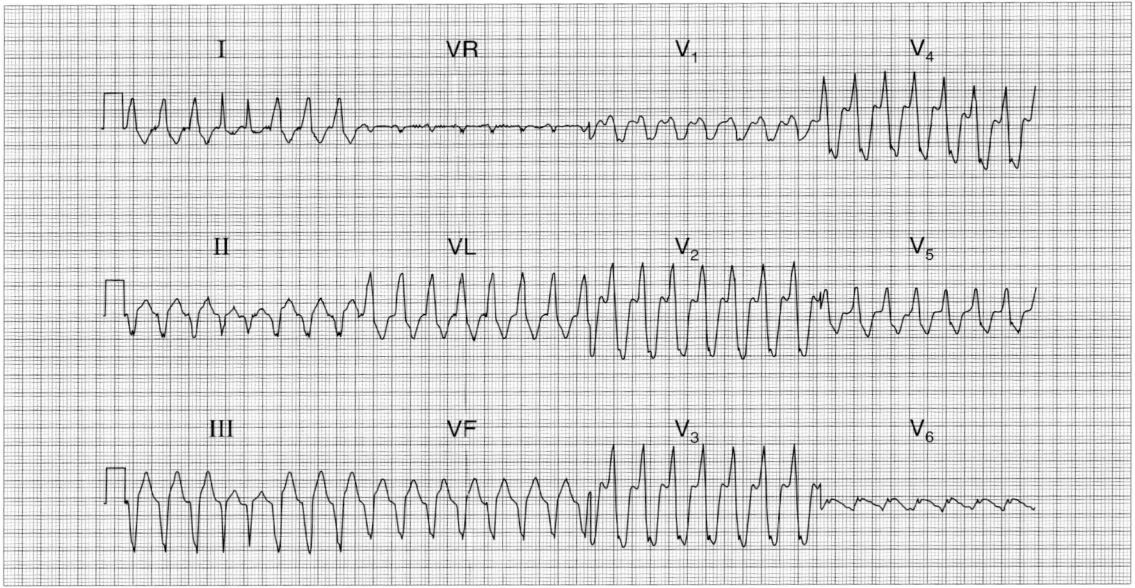

ECG 108 A 70-year-old woman, admitted to hospital because of increasing heart failure of uncertain cause, collapsed and was found to have a very rapid pulse and a low blood pressure. This is her ECG. She recovered spontaneously. What is this rhythm, and what would you do?

ANSWER 108

The ECG shows:

- Broad complex tachycardia at about 180/min
- No P waves visible
- Left axis
- QRS duration about 140 ms
- The fourth and fifth QRS complexes are narrow
- QRS complexes are probably concordant (in the chest leads all point upwards) though it is difficult to be certain

Clinical interpretation

Broad complex tachycardias may be ventricular, supraventricular with bundle branch block, or may be due to a Wolff–Parkinson–White syndrome. We have no ECG from this patient recorded when she was in sinus rhythm, which is always the most helpful thing in deciding between these possibilities. The complexes are not very wide, which would be consistent with a supraventricular origin with aberrant conduction, but the left axis and (probable) concordance point to ventricular tachycardia. The key is the two narrow complexes near the beginning of the record: these are slightly early and are probably capture beats. They indicate that with an early supraventricular beat the conducting system can function normally; by implication, the broad complexes must be due to ventricular tachycardia.

What to do

An elderly patient with heart failure is more likely to have ischaemic disease than anything else, but all ther possible causes of heart failure must be considered. The sudden onset of an arrhythmia could be due to a myocardial infarction. Pulmonary emboli can cause sudden arrhythmias, though these are more often supraventricular than ventricular. It is important to consider whether this rhythm change is related to treatment, either because of an electrolyte imbalance or the pro-arrhythmic effect of a drug the patient is taking.

Summary ★★★
Ventricular tachycardia.

ME See p. 72
IP See p. 192

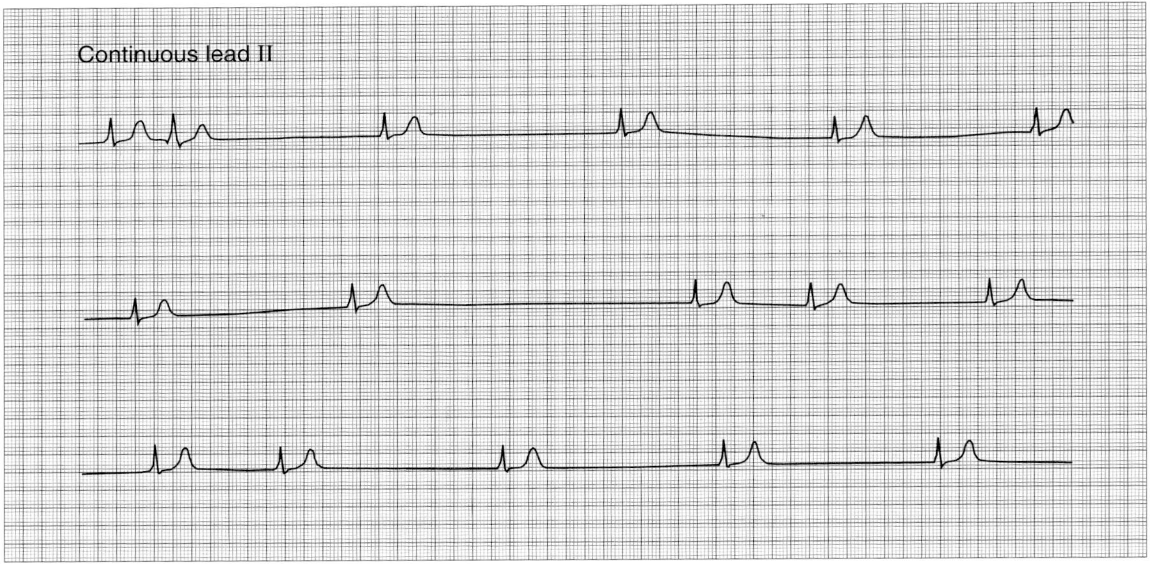

ECG 109 This is a continuous rhythm strip (lead II) from a 25-year-old man who complained of episodes of fast, regular, palpitations associated with breathlessness and dizziness. There were no abnormalities on examination other than a slow and irregular pulse, and apart from the rhythm shown here, the ECG was normal. What is the diagnosis and how can his problem be treated?

ANSWER 109

The ECG shows:

- Variable QRS rate (16–60/min)
- No P waves
- No irregular baseline to suggest atrial fibrillation
- As far as can be ascertained from the rhythm strip, normal QRS complexes and T waves

Clinical interpretation
This is the 'sick sinus syndrome' or 'sinoatrial disease'. The record shows a 'silent atrium' with a variable junctional escape rhythm. The palpitations described by the patient are probably due to a paroxysmal supraventricular tachycardia, so he probably has the 'bradycardia-tachycardia' variant of sinoatrial disease.

What to do
Ambulatory ECG tape-recording will confirm the cause of the patient's palpitations. Even though his bradycardia is asymptomatic, he will need a permanent pacemaker because anti-arrhythmic agents given for the tachycardia may make his bradycardia worse.

Summary ★★★
Sinoatrial disease with a 'silent atrium' and junctional escape.

IP See p. 199

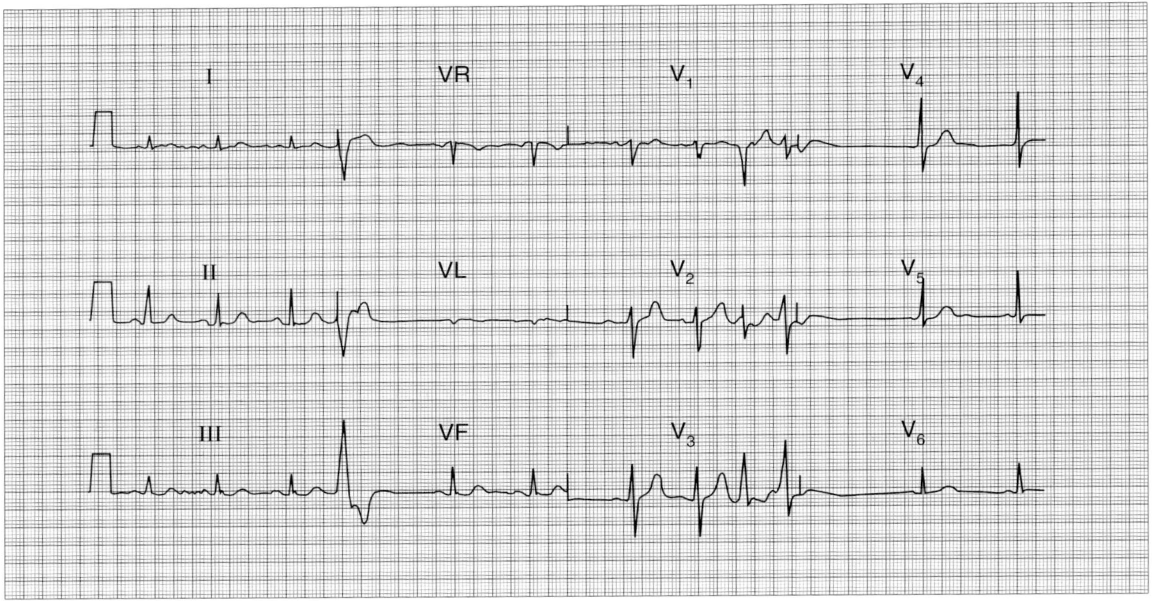

ECG 110 This ECG was recorded from an 80-year-old man during a routine preoperative assessment. What does it show? What are the implications for surgery?

ANSWER 110

The ECG shows:

- Sinus rhythm with ventricular extrasystoles
- Ventricular extrasystoles are of two types, seen best in lead V_3
- Normal axis
- Normal QRS complexes
- ST segments and T waves are normal

Clinical interpretation
Sinus rhythm, with multifocal ventricular extrasystoles but otherwise normal.

What to do
In large groups of patients, ventricular extrasystoles are correlated with heart disease of all types. In individuals, however, extrasystoles may well occur in a perfectly normal heart – indeed virtually everyone has extrasystoles at times. Ventricular extrasystoles become more common with increasing age, and this patient is 80 years old. In the absence of symptoms or clinical signs suggesting cardiovascular disease, the extrasystoles do not have any great significance and should not materially affect the patient's fitness for surgery. They should not be treated.

Summary ★
Sinus rhythm with multifocal ventricular extrasystoles.

ME See p. 64
IP See p. 104

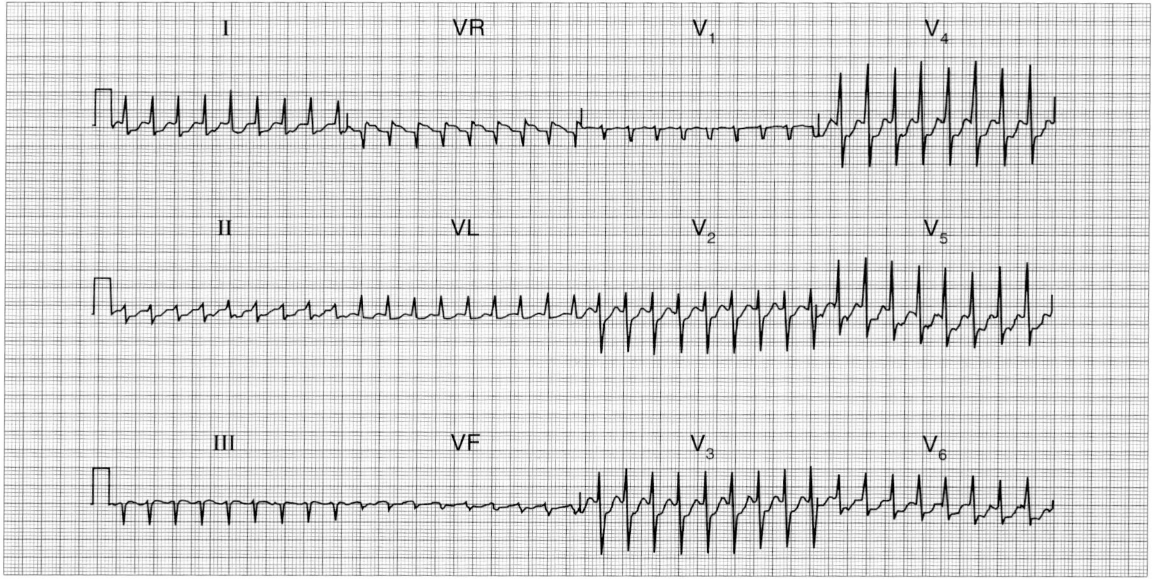

ECG 111 A 50-year-old man was admitted to hospital as an emergency with chest pain; he was not aware of a rapid heart rate. He had had several episodes of pain that appeared to be due to ischaemia, but these had no clear relationship with exertion. Shortly after this ECG was recorded, his heart rate suddenly slowed and his ECG was then normal. What does this record show, and what would you do?

ANSWER 111

The ECG shows:

- Narrow complex tachycardia, rate about 200/min
- No P waves
- Normal axis
- Normal QRS complexes
- Horizontal ST segment depression, most marked in lead V_4

Clinical interpretation
Narrow complex tachycardia without P waves – atrioventricular re-entry (junctional) tachycardia. Ischaemic ST segment depression, accounting for his pain.

What to do
Not all patients with a paroxysmal tachycardia complain of palpitations; this patient's recurrent chest pain may well have been due to this arrhythmia. He should be taught the methods of inducing vagal activity, but prophylactic drug therapy will be needed: a beta-blocker or verapamil should be tried first. Electrophysiological investigation, with a view to ablating an abnormal pathway, may be needed.

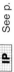

Summary ★
Junctional tachycardia with ischaemia.

ME See pp. 72 and 102

IP See p. 44

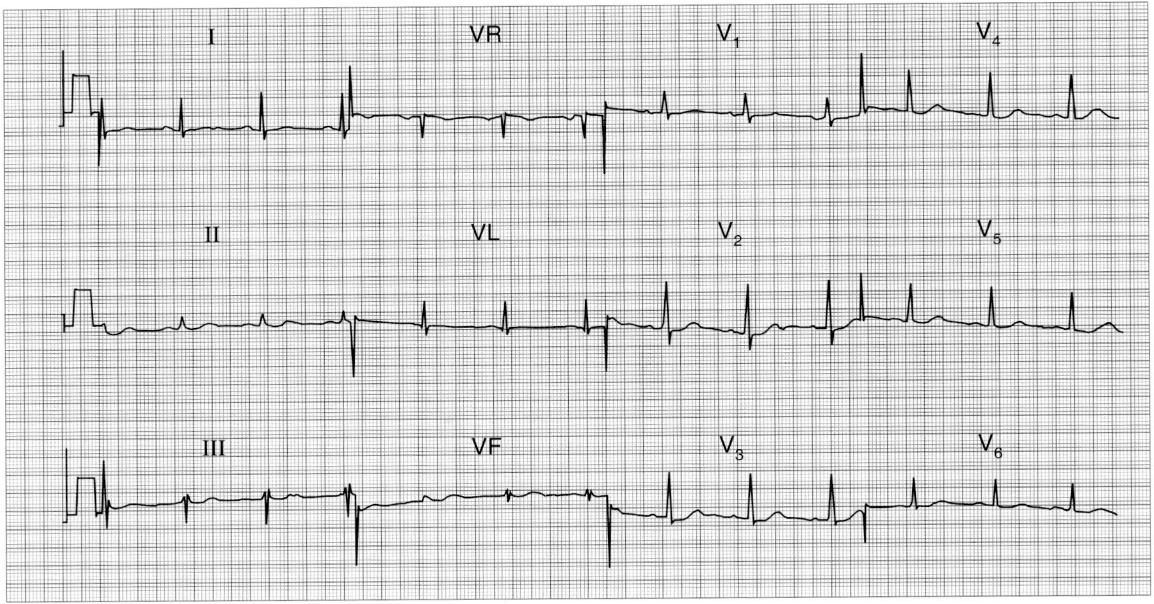

ECG 112 A 40-year-old man is seen in the out-patient department with a history that suggests a myocardial infarction 3 weeks previously. There are no abnormalities on examination, and this is his ECG. There are two possible explanations for the abnormality it shows, though only one of these explains his history. What is the likely diagnosis?

ANSWER 112

The ECG shows:

- Sinus rhythm
- Normal axis
- Dominant R waves in lead V_1
- Non-specific T wave flattening in leads I, VL

Clinical interpretation

The dominant R waves in lead V_1 might indicate right ventricular hypertrophy, but there are none of the other features that would be associated with this – right axis deviation, and T wave inversion in leads V_1, V_2 and possibly V_3. The changes are therefore probably due to a posterior myocardial infarction, which would fit the history of chest pain 3 weeks previously.

What to do

It is important not to miss a diagnosis of pulmonary embolism. The patient should be re-examined to ensure that there is no clinical evidence of right ventricular hypertrophy. A chest X-ray examination with a lateral view should be arranged, and an echocardiogram may be helpful.

Summary ★★
Probable posterior myocardial infarction.

ME See p. 96

IP See p. 250

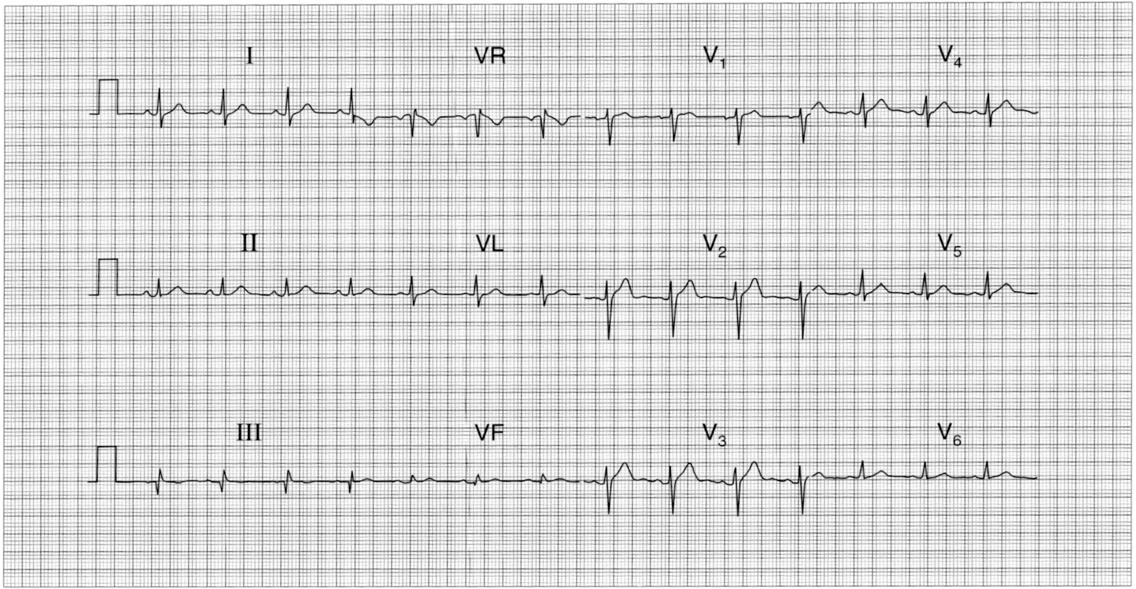

ECG 113 This ECG was recorded from a 60-year-old man with no symptoms, who wanted a private pilot's licence. Is it normal? How could you convince the licensing authority?

ANSWER 113

The ECG shows:

- Sinus rhythm
- Normal conduction
- Normal axis
- Q wave in lead III but not in lead VF
- Inverted T wave in lead III but not in lead VF

Clinical interpretation

A Q wave and an inverted T wave in lead III, but not in lead VF, is a normal variant. If lead III is recorded with the patient taking a deep breath in, the changes will usually normalize as shown on the right.

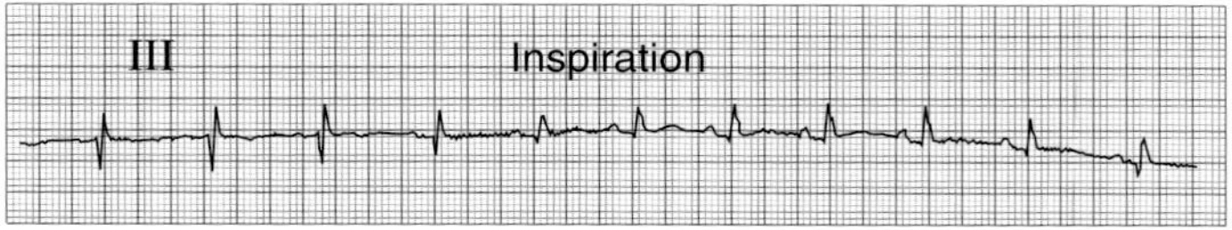

Summary ★★

Normal record.

IP See p. 80

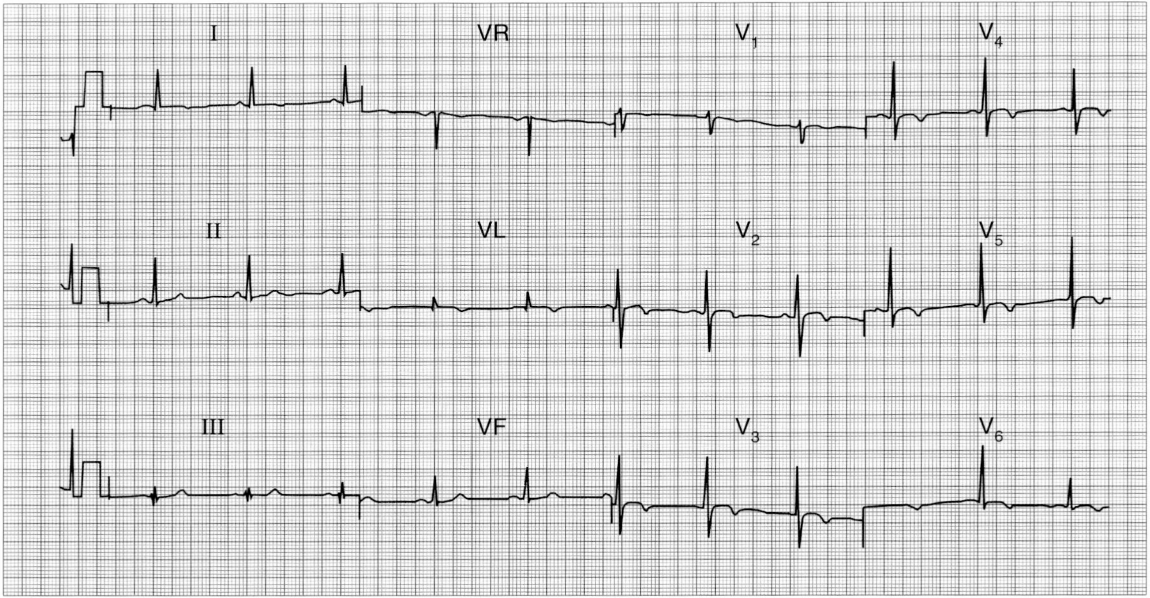

ECG 114 This ECG was recorded from a 55-year-old black woman who had been complaining for several years of chest pain, and who was admitted to hospital with persistent pain that was not characteristic of ischaemia. How would you have managed her?

ANSWER 114

The ECG shows:

- Sinus rhythm
- Normal axis
- Normal QRS complexes
- T wave inversion in leads I, VL, V_2–V_6

Clinical interpretation

With this history a non-Q wave anterolateral infarction has to be the first diagnosis, but T wave 'abnormalities' are common in black people, and this ECG could be normal.

What to do

In this patient an infarction was excluded when the cardiac enzyme levels were found to be normal. An exercise test was performed, but was limited by breathlessness without further ECG change. A coronary angiogram was completely normal.

Summary ★★★

Widespread T wave 'abnormalities,' normal in a black woman.

ME See p. 112

IP See p. 89

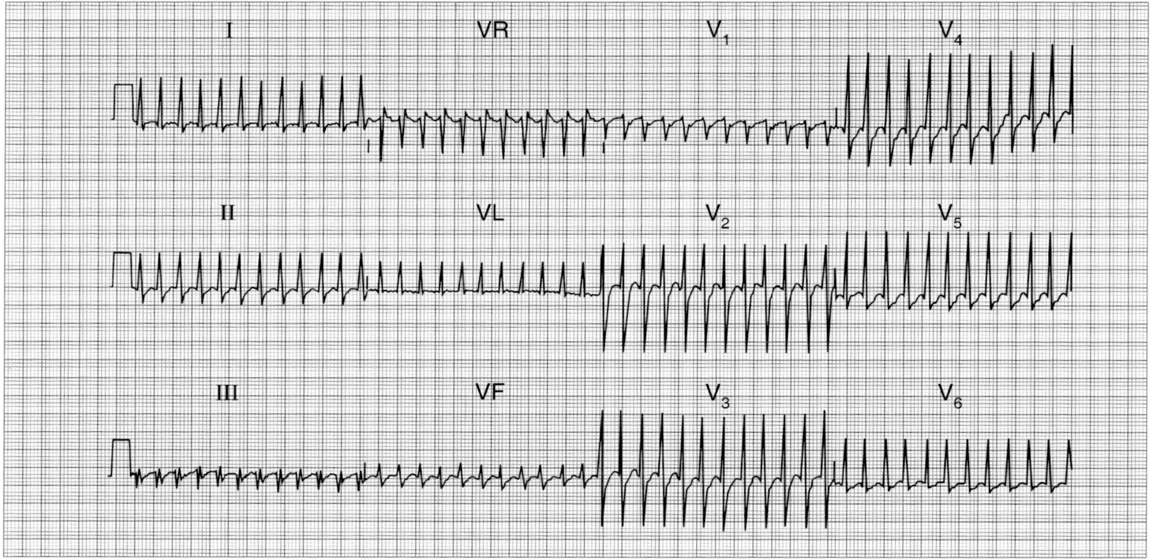

ECG 115 A 50-year-old man, who had complained of attacks of dizziness and palpitations for several years, collapsed at work and was brought to the A & E department. He was cold and clammy. His heart rate was rapid and his blood pressure was unrecordable. There were signs of left ventricular failure. This is his ECG. What does it show and what would you do?

ANSWER 115

The ECG shows:

- Narrow-complex tachycardia, rate 300/min
- No definite P waves
- Normal QRS complexes
- Horizontal ST segment depression in lead V_5

Clinical interpretation

A regular narrow-complex tachycardia at 300/min probably represents atrial flutter with 1:1 conduction (i.e. each atrial activation causes ventricular activation).

What to do

The cardiovascular collapse results from the rapid heart rate, with a loss of diastolic filling. Carotid sinus pressure may temporarily increase the degree of block and establish the diagnosis, but it is unlikely to convert atrial flutter to sinus rhythm. Intravenous adenosine is likely to have the same effect. A patient who is haemodynamically compromised by a tachycardia should be treated with immediate DC cardioversion.

Summary ★★

Probable atrial flutter with 1:1 conduction.

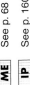

ME See p. 68

IP See p. 160

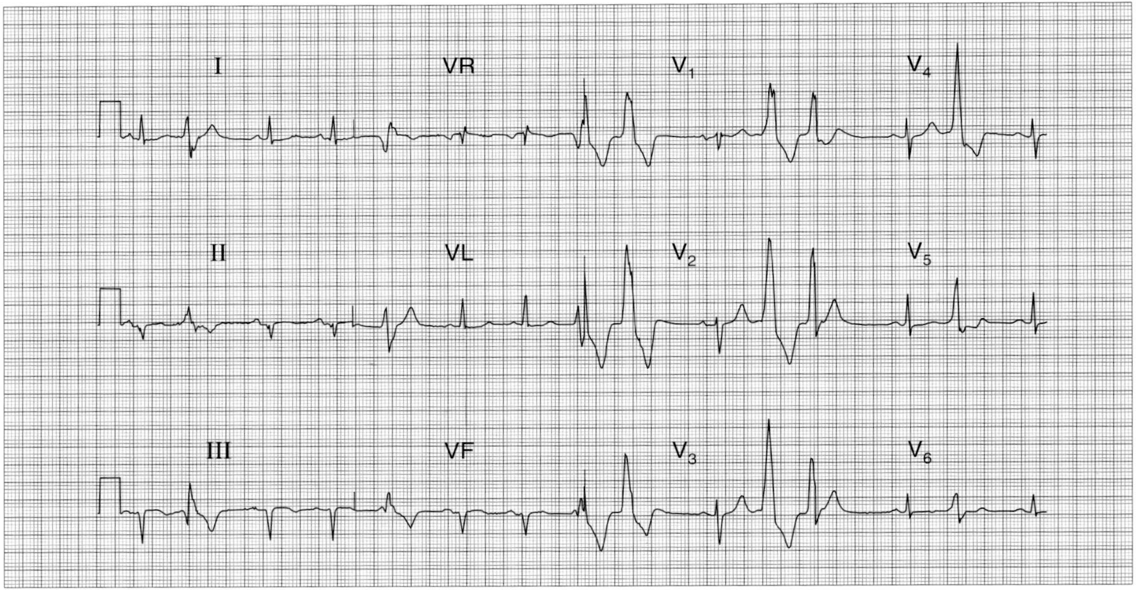

ECG 116 A 70-year-old man, who had had angina for several years, began to complain of dizzy attacks. This is his ECG. What does it show and what would you do?

ANSWER 116

The ECG shows:

- Sinus rhythm with frequent multifocal ventricular extrasystoles
- Normal PR interval
- Normal axis
- Q waves in leads II, III, VF
- T waves flattened or inverted in leads II, III, V_5–V_6

Clinical interpretation
The ECG shows a probable old inferior myocardial infarction, which accounts for his angina. Ventricular extrasystoles are of themselves usually not important, but in a patient complaining of dizzy attacks, ventricular extrasystoles that are frequent and multifocal may be causing haemodynamic impairment.

What to do
It would be worth recording an ambulatory ECG to see if the patient is having runs of ventricular tachycardia, but the extrasystoles probably do need suppressing. Sotalol would be the first drug to try, and then amiodarone.

Summary ★★
Old inferior myocardial infarction and frequent multifocal ventricular extrasystoles.

ME See p. 96
IP See p. 154

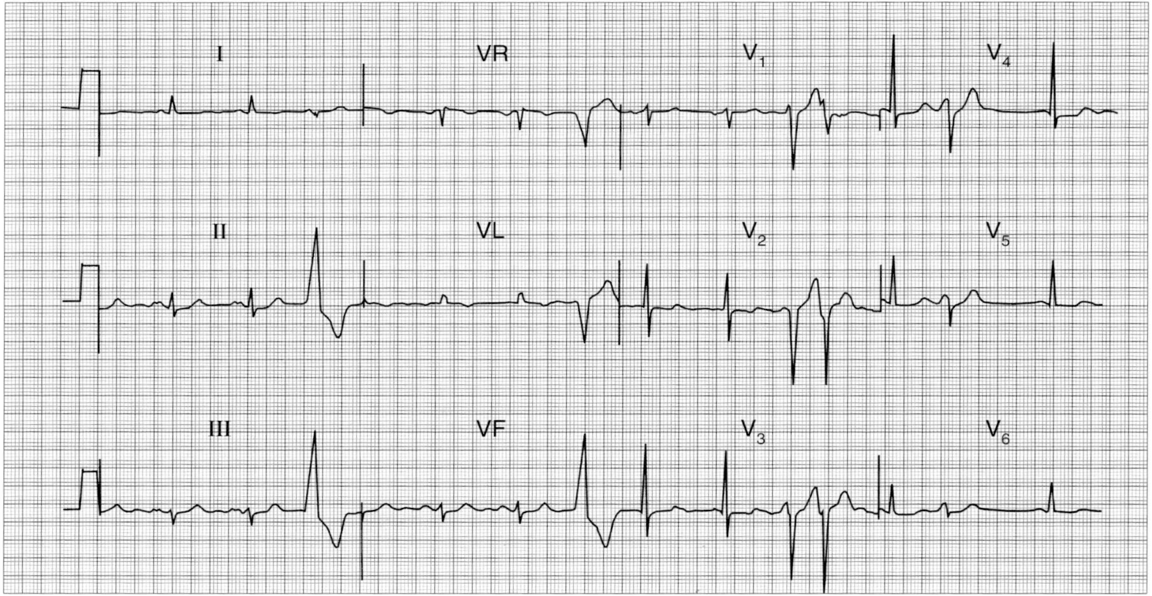

ECG 117 This ECG was recorded from a 50-year-old woman who complained of breathlessness and palpitations. What physical signs would you look for, and what is the next stage in her management?

ANSWER 117

The ECG shows:

- Sinus rhythm with ventricular extrasystoles
- Broad notched P waves, best seen in leads II, III, VF
- Normal axis
- Normal QRS complexes
- Biphasic T waves in leads V_2, V_3; inverted T waves in lead VL

Clinical interpretation

The broad P waves suggest left atrial hypertrophy. There is nothing to suggest left ventricular hypertrophy, so mitral stenosis must be considered. Ventricular extrasystoles may explain the palpitations, but if the patient has mitral stenosis she may be having episodes of atrial fibrillation. The cause of the T wave changes is not clear and may be ischaemia.

What to do

Look for the tapping apex beat, the loud first sound, the opening snap and the mid-diastolic murmur that are characteristic of mitral stenosis. Echocardiography will probably be helpful, and ambulatory ECG tape-recording may be necessary to identify the cause of the palpitations. Treatments to be considered if she has mitral valve disease and atrial fibrillation are digoxin, anticoagulants, and mitral valve surgery.

If the breathlessness turns out to be due to poor left ventricular function, an angiotensin-converting enzyme inhibitor is needed.

Summary ★★
Sinus rhythm with ventricular extrasystoles, left atrial hypertrophy and possible ischaemia.

ME See p. 89
IP See p. 318

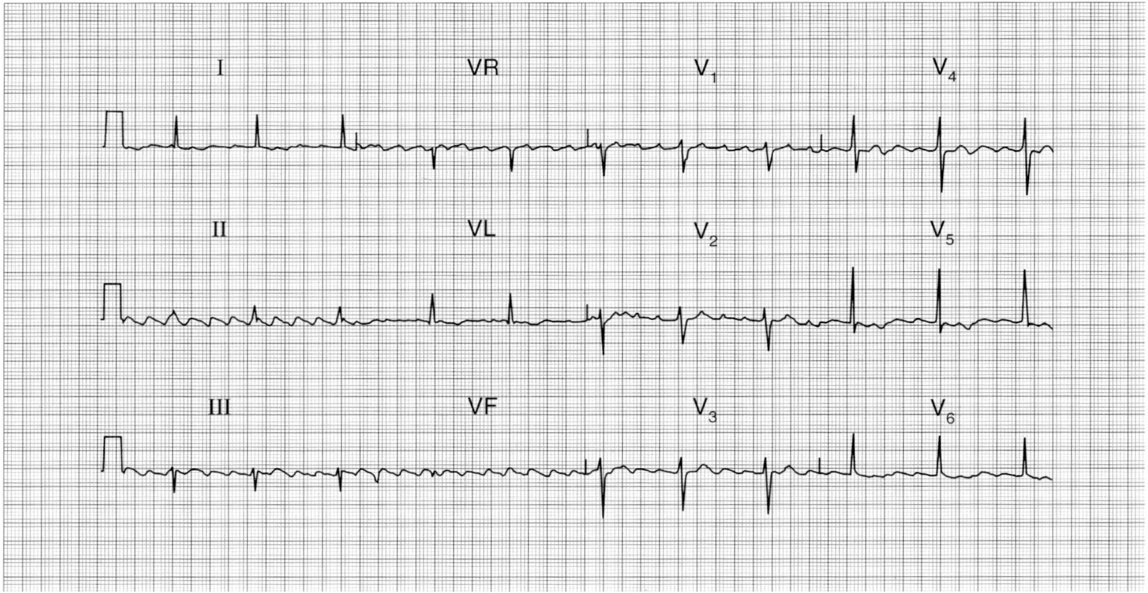

ECG 118 A 60-year-old man who complains of ankle swelling is found to have a regular pulse, a blood pressure of 115/70, an enlarged heart, and signs of congestive cardiac failure. This is his ECG. What does it show? He is untreated – how would you manage him?

ANSWER 118

The ECG shows:

- Atrial flutter with 4:1 block
- Normal axis
- Slight QRS widening
- T waves are difficult to identify but at least in lead VL are inverted

Clinical interpretation

Atrial flutter with stable 4:1 conduction explains why the heart is clinically regular. The slight QRS widening is non-specific. There is no evidence of a previous infarction or of ventricular hypertrophy; the T wave inversion could be ischaemic, but may well be due to a dilated cardiomyopathy.

What to do

An echocardiogram will show if he has a dilated left ventricle, if there is general left ventricular dysfunction or if there are parts of the left ventricle that contract well and others that do not, which would suggest ischaemia.

Atrial flutter is a difficult rhythm to treat: if the heart is enlarged it is unlikely that sinus rhythm can be restored either by drugs or by DC cardioversion, and if the block is stable (as appears here) it may be best left alone. Digoxin must be used cautiously in case it induces a higher degree of block and bradycardia. The heart failure should be treated with an angiotensin-converting enzyme inhibitor and a diuretic.

This patient had an alcoholic dilated cardiomyopathy.

Summary ★
Atrial flutter with 4:1 block.

ME See p. 68

IP See pp. 160 and 230

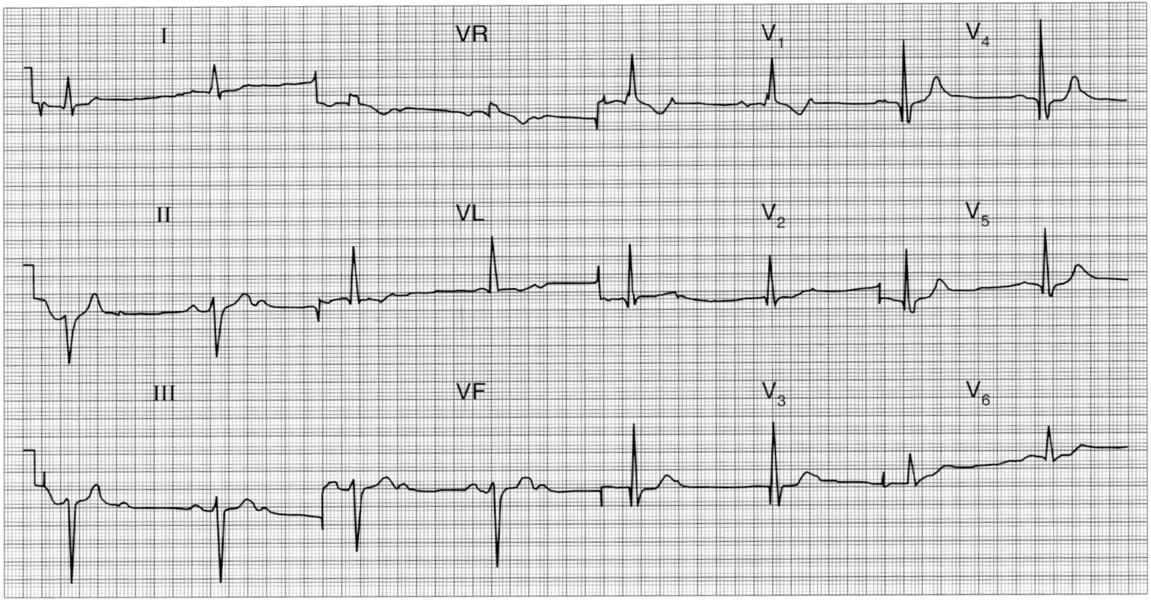

ECG 119 A 70-year-old man is sent to the out-patient department because of attacks of dizziness. What abnormalities does his ECG show, and what treatment is needed?

ANSWER 119

The ECG shows:

- Sinus rhythm
- Second degree (2:1) heart block
- Left axis deviation
- Right bundle branch block

Clinical interpretation

Left axis deviation is due to left anterior fascicular block (left anterior hemiblock). Since right bundle branch block is present, intra-ventricular conduction depends on the posterior fascicle. The presence of second degree block suggests that conduction in this fascicle is already impaired or that there may be impaired conduction in the bundle of His.

What to do

This patient's attacks of dizziness may be due to the slow heart rate demonstrated in this ECG, or may represent intermittent periods of complete block with an even slower rate and Stokes–Adams attacks. Permanent pacing is urgently needed and the patient should be admitted to the hospital from the out-patient department.

Summary ★★★
Second degree (2:1) block, left anterior hemiblock, and right bundle branch block (trifascicular block).

ME See pp. 31 and 48

IP See p. 21

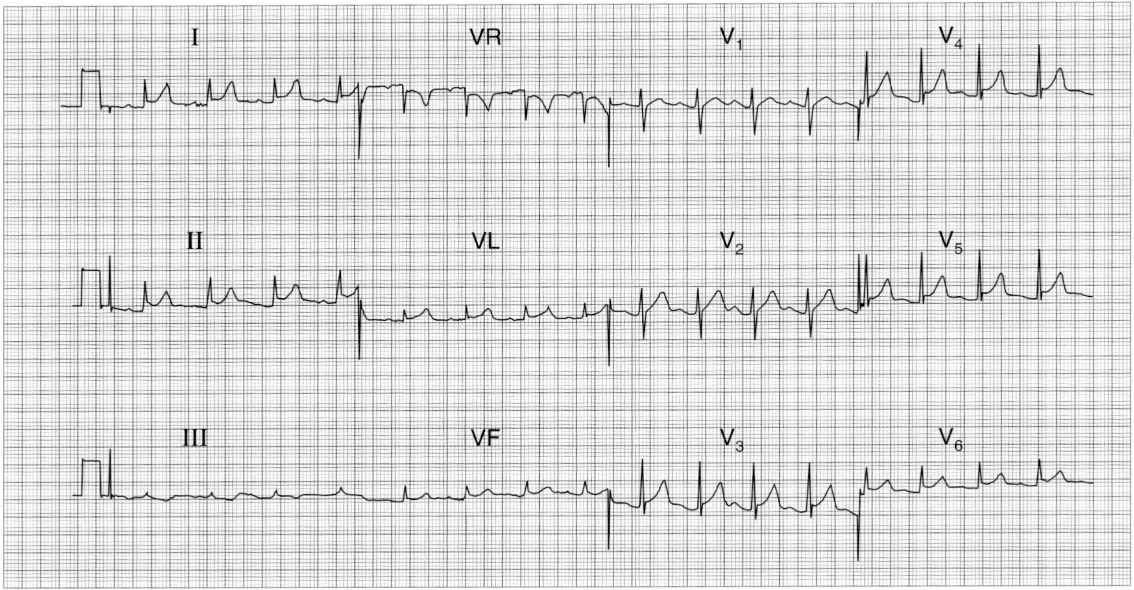

ECG 120 This ECG was recorded from a 30-year-old man admitted with severe central chest pain. He was a heavy smoker and had a bad family history of ischaemic heart disease. The physical examination was reported to be normal. What do you think is going on?

ANSWER 120

The ECG shows:

- Sinus rhythm, rate 100/min
- Normal conduction
- Normal axis
- Normal QRS complexes
- Raised ST segments in leads I, II, VL, V_3–V_6
- 'High take off' ST segment in leads V_3–V_5
- T wave inversion in lead III

Clinical interpretation

In a patient with chest pain and risk factors for a myocardial infarction, an infarction must obviously be the first diagnosis. The raised ST segments on this ECG could support this diagnosis. However, the patient is very young to have an infarction. The 'high take-off' ST segments in leads V_3–V_5 (raised ST segment following an S wave) are a normal variant. The other raised ST segments could well be due to pericarditis.

What to do

The patient should be examined lying flat, because this gives the best chance of hearing a pericardial friction rub – and this is what was found here. The pericarditis could, of course, be due to an infarction, but repeated ECGs showed no development of an infarction pattern, and the raised ST segments persisted for several days. A diagnosis of viral pericarditis was eventually made.

Summary ★★

ST segment elevation, partly 'high take-off' and partly due to pericarditis.

ME See p. 100

IP See pp. 82 and 298

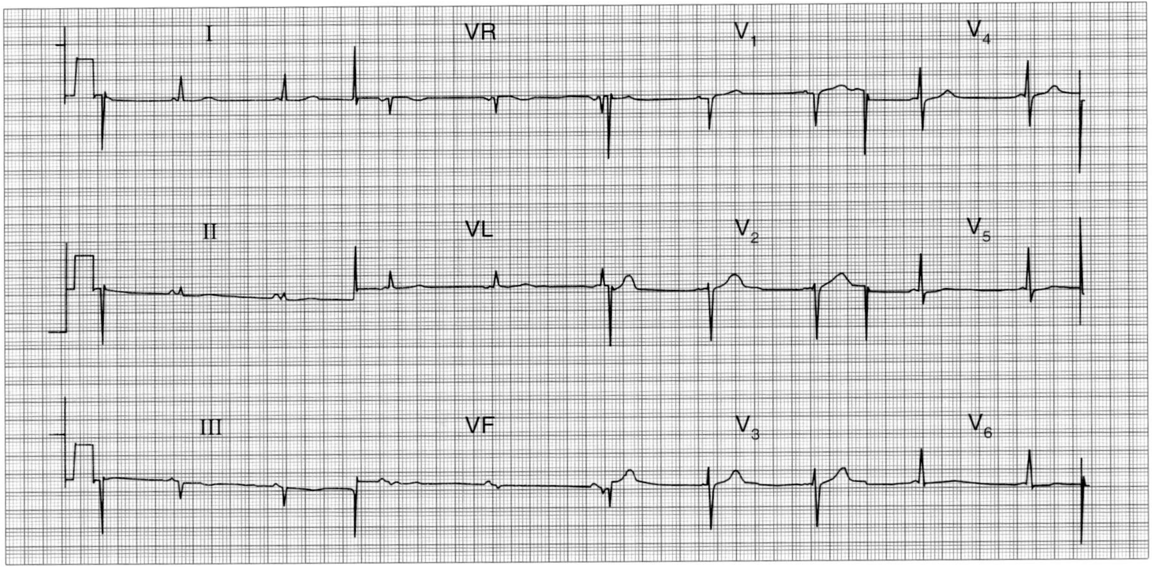

ECG 121 An 18-year-old student complains of occasional attacks of palpitations. These start suddenly without provocation; the heart beat seems regular and is 'too fast to count'. During attacks she does not feel dizzy or breathless, and the palpitations stop suddenly after a few seconds. Physical examination is normal, and this is her ECG. What is the diagnosis and what advice would you give?

ANSWER 121

The ECG shows:

- Sinus rhythm
- Very short PR interval
- Normal axis
- Normal QRS complexes and T waves

Clinical interpretation

This is the Lown–Ganong–Levine syndrome. Unlike the Wolff–Parkinson–White syndrome, in which there is an accessory pathway separate from the atrioventricular node and His bundle, in the Lown–Ganong–Levine syndrome there is a bypass close to the atrioventricular node connecting the left atrium and the His bundle. In the Wolff–Parkinson–White syndrome the QRS complex shows an early delta wave, but in the Lown–Ganong–Levine syndrome the QRS complex is normal.

What to do

Ambulatory ECG tape-recording may confirm the diagnosis if attacks are frequent enough. Infrequent and short-lived attacks such as this patient describes are not dangerous, but she should be taught vagal-stimulating procedures such as Valsalva's manoeuvre and carotid sinus pressure. An electrophysiological study and ablation of the abnormal tract may be necessary.

Summary ★★★
Lown–Ganong–Levine syndrome.

IP See pp. 40 and 127

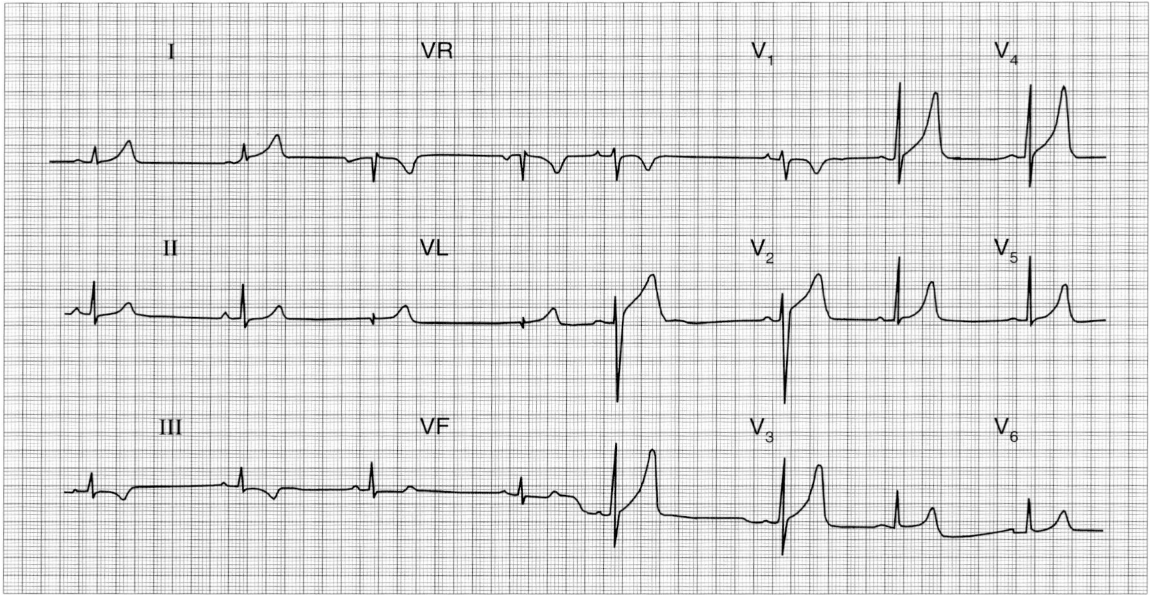

ECG 122 This ECG was recorded from a 37-year-old man admitted to hospital for a routine orthopaedic operation. The anaesthetist asks for comments.

ANSWER 122

The ECG shows:

- Sinus rhythm, 45/min
- Normal axis
- Normal QRS complexes
- Inverted T waves in lead III and ST segment depression in lead VF
- Peaked T waves in the anterior leads

Clinical interpretation

Provided the patient is not taking a beta-blocker, the slow heart rate is probably a reflection of physical fitness. Inverted T waves in lead III, and the downward-sloping ST segments in lead VF, are probably normal. Peaked T waves are characteristic of hyperkalaemia, and are sometimes described as 'hyperacute' in ischaemia. However, when as large as this – and particularly when the patient is asymptomatic – peaked T waves are nearly always perfectly normal.

What to do

Ensure that the patient has no cardiac symptoms, and check his electrolyte levels pre-operatively.

Summary ★★★
Normal ECG.

IP See p. 91

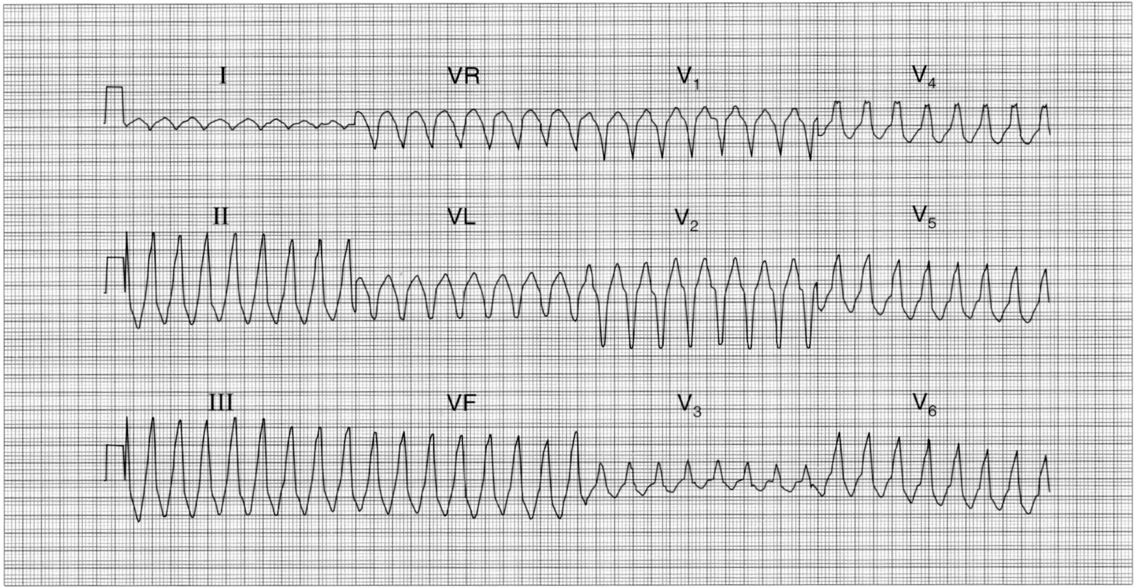

ECG 123 A 30-year-old man, who had had attacks of palpitations for several years, was seen during an attack, and this ECG was recorded. He was breathless and his blood pressure was unrecordable. What does the ECG show and how should he be treated?

ANSWER 123

The ECG shows:

- Broad complex tachycardia at 200/min
- No P waves visible
- Right axis
- QRS duration 200ms
- QRS complex shows no concordance; left bundle branch block (LBBB) pattern

Clinical interpretation

A broad complex tachycardia like this is probably of ventricular origin, but here features against this rhythm being ventricular tachycardia are the right axis and the lack of concordance in the QRS complexes (i.e. the complexes point downwards in leads V_1 and V_2 and upwards in the other chest leads). However, the combination of right axis and an LBBB pattern in a broad complex tachycardia suggests that the origin is in the right ventricular outflow tract.

What to do

Any patient with an arrhythmia and evidence of haemodynamic compromise (in this case, breathlessness and a very low blood pressure) needs immediate cardioversion. While preparations are being made, it would be reasonable to try intravenous lignocaine or amiodarone. Once the arrhythmia has been corrected an electrophysiological study is needed, for right ventricular outflow tract tachycardia is the one variety of ventricular tachycardia that should be amenable to ablation therapy.

Summary ★★★

Ventricular tachycardia, probably originating in the right ventricular outflow tract.

ME See p. 75

IP See p. 195

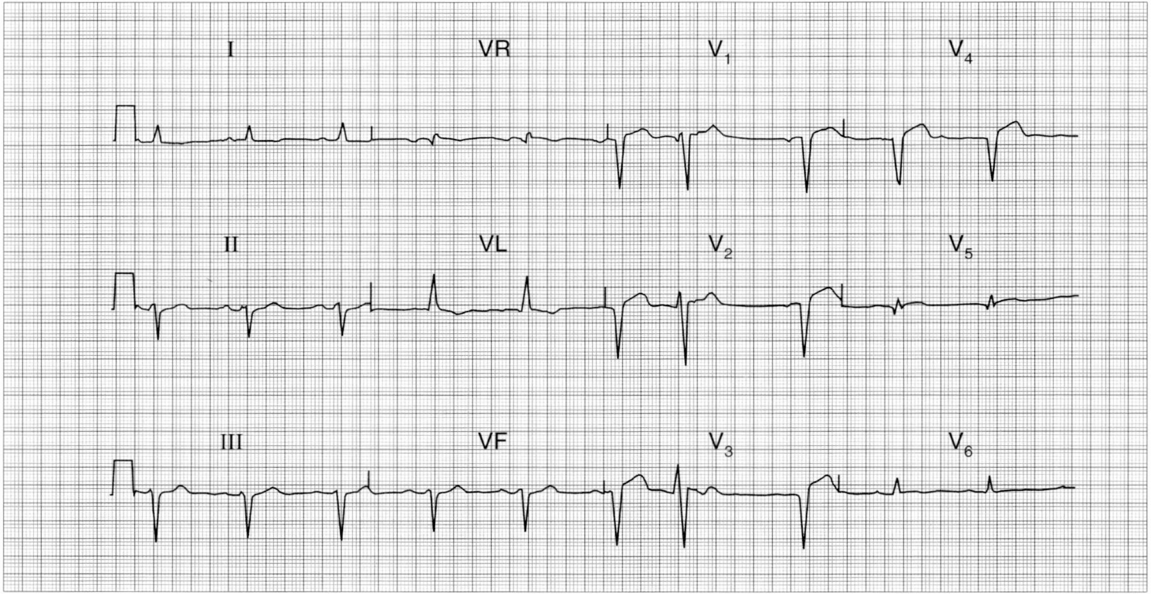

ECG 124 This ECG was recorded from a 75-year-old man with heart failure. He did not complain of chest pain. There are three main abnormalities. How should he be treated?

ANSWER 124

The ECG shows:

- Sinus rhythm with one ventricular extrasystole
- Left axis deviation
- Slight widening of the QRS complexes
- Q waves in leads V_2–V_5
- Raised ST segments in the anterior leads
- Inverted T wave in lead VL; flattened T waves in leads I, V_6

Clinical interpretation

A 'silent' anterior infarction of uncertain age has caused left anterior hemiblock, which explains the left axis deviation and widening of the QRS complexes. The lateral T wave changes are presumably due to ischaemia.

What to do

Ventricular extrasystoles should not be treated, and left anterior hemiblock is not an indication for pacing. In the absence of pain, the anterior infarction cannot be assumed to be new, so thrombolysis should not be given. He needs an angiotensin-converting enzyme inhibitor and diuretic.

Summary ★★

Left anterior hemiblock and anterior infarction of uncertain age; one ventricular extrasystole.

ME See pp. 46 and 95

IP See p. 18

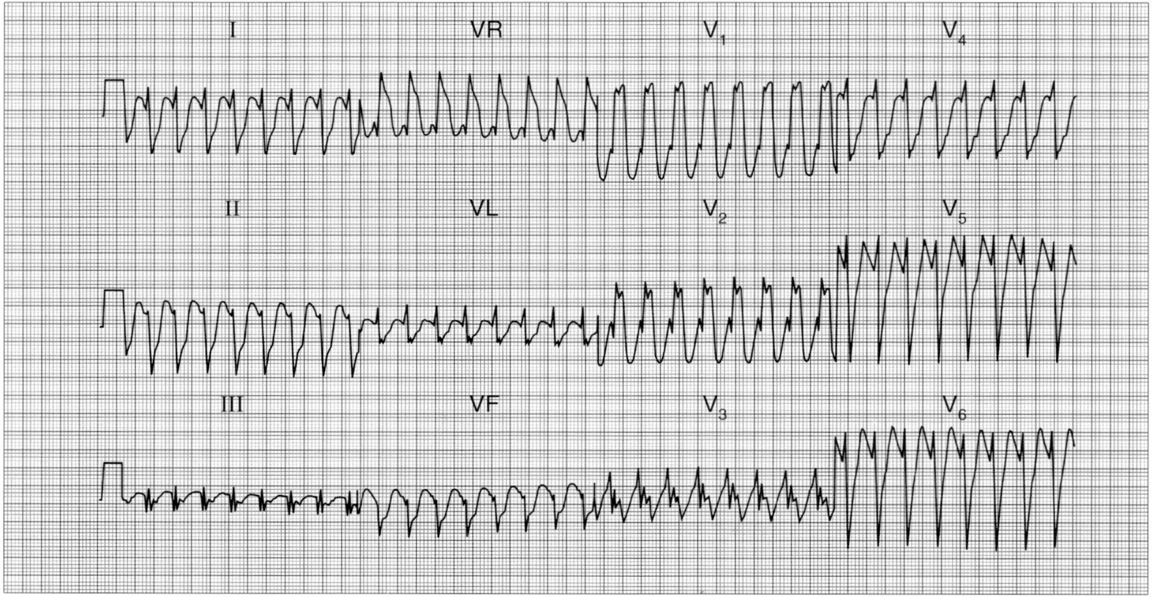

ECG 125 A 35-year-old woman, who had had palpitations for many years without any diagnosis being made, was eventually seen in the A & E department during an attack. She looked well and was not in heart failure, and her blood pressure was 120/70. This is her ECG. What is the rhythm, and what would you do?

ANSWER 125

The ECG shows:

- Broad-complex tachycardia (QRS complex 200 ms), rate nearly 200/min
- No P waves visible
- Right axis deviation
- Right bundle branch block pattern
- In lead V_1, the R^1 peak is higher than the R peak

Clinical interpretation

The problem here is to distinguish a supraventricular tachycardia with bundle branch block from ventricular tachycardia. The clinical history is not helpful, nor is the fact that the patient is haemodynamically stable. The combination of right axis deviation, right bundle branch block and the R^1 peak being higher than the R peak make it likely that this is a supraventricular tachycardia with right bundle branch block rather than ventricular tachycardia. However, the very broad QRS complex (>140 ms) would favour a ventricular origin for the arrhythmia.

What to do

Carotid sinus massage. If this has no effect try intravenous adenosine, and if this is ineffective try intravenous lignocaine.

Summary ★★★

Broad-complex tachycardia with right bundle branch block pattern, probably supraventricular in origin.

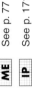

ME See p. 77

IP See p. 171

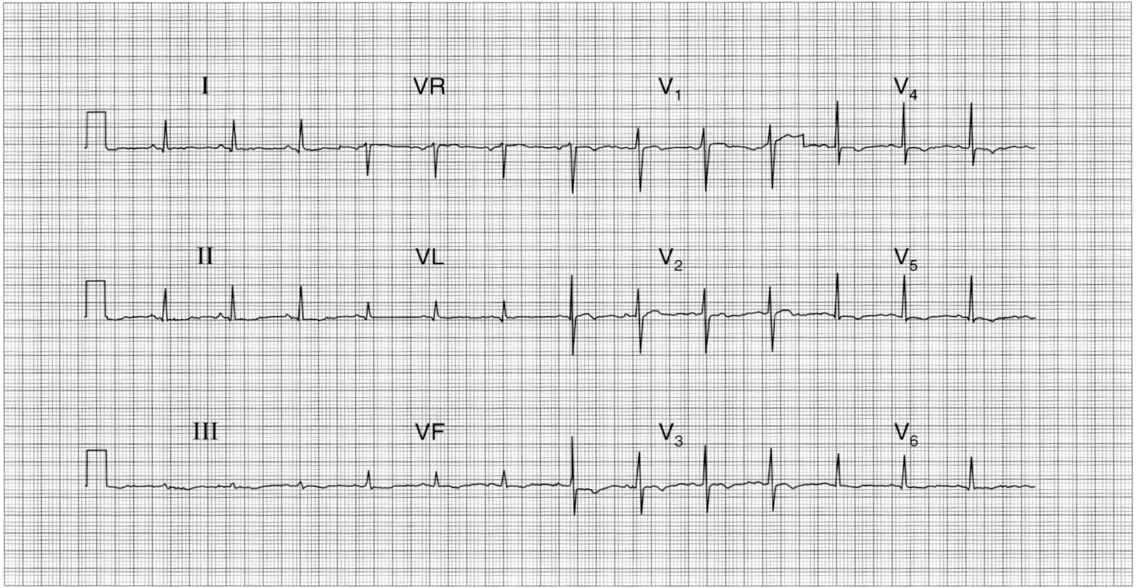

ECG 126 This ECG was recorded as part of the routine investigation of a 40-year-old man who was admitted following a first seizure. He was unconscious, had a stiff neck, and bilateral extensor plantar responses. His heart was clinically normal. What do you think has happened?

ANSWER 126

This ECG shows:

- Sinus rhythm, rate 80/min
- Normal PR interval and QRS duration
- Normal axis
- Normal QRS complexes
- ST depression in lead II
- T wave inversion in leads III, VF, V_4–V_6

Clinical interpretation

The appearances here are suggestive of an anterior non-Q wave myocardial infarction, but this does not correspond with the clinical picture.

What to do

It is possible that this patient had a myocardial infarction which caused a cerebrovascular accident because of an arrhythmia, or because of a cerebral embolus, and that the cerebrovascular accident caused the seizure. The unconsciousness and the bilateral extensor plantar responses could simply be post-ictal. However, such a sequence would not explain the stiff neck, which would seem to point to either a subarachnoid haemorrhage or meningitis. Changes like those on this ECG are common in subarachnoid haemorrhage, probably because of intense coronary vasospasm resulting from catecholamine release. Measurements of the blood troponin level are unlikely to help differentiate between a primarily cardiac and a primarily neurological event. This patient did indeed have a subarachnoid haemorrhage, and the ECG eventually returned to normal.

Summary ★★★
Anterior and inferior T wave inversion due to subarachnoid haemorrhage.

IP See p. 382

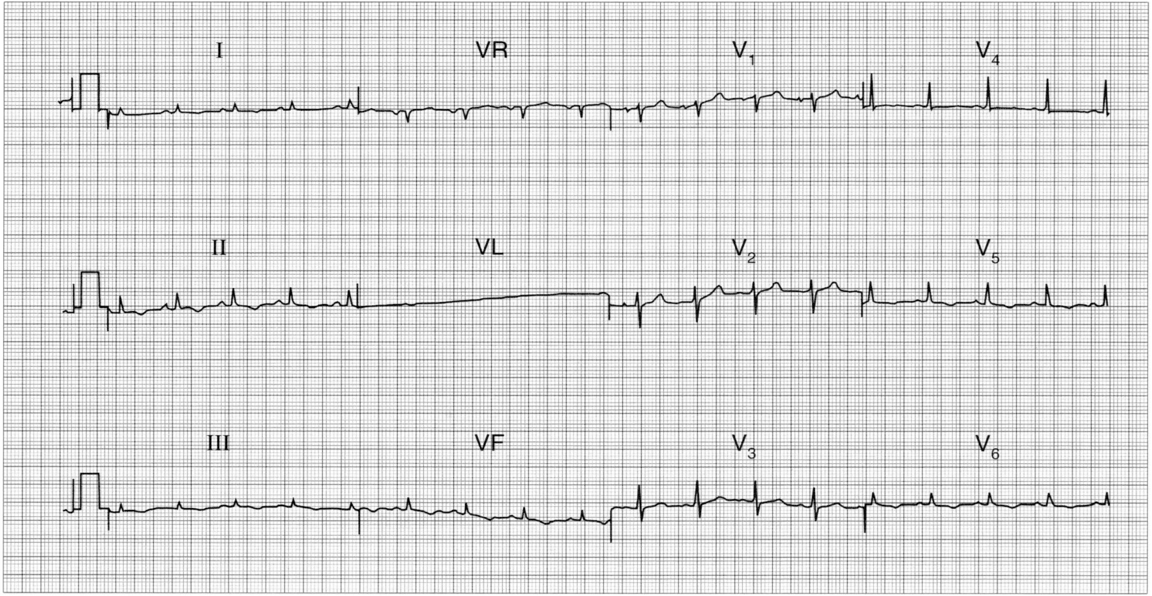

ECG 127 A 70-year-old man with lung cancer is admitted to hospital with abdominal pain and ankle swelling. He has a raised jugular venous pressure, a tender and distended liver, and marked peripheral oedema. Does this ECG help with the diagnosis and what might you need to do?

ANSWER 127

The ECG shows:

- Sinus rhythm
- Normal axis
- Normal width but generally small QRS complexes
- T wave inversion in leads I, II, III, VF, V_5–V_6

Clinical interpretation

Small QRS complexes are seen with a pericardial effusion, and sometimes in patients with chronic lung disease. The widespread T wave changes would be consistent with pericardial disease. There is nothing in this record to suggest pulmonary disease.

What to do

The physical findings and the ECG would fit with a pericardial effusion associated with malignancy. You should look carefully at the jugular venous pressure to see if it rises with inspiration, indicating pericardial tamponade. Echocardiography is essential, and if there is evidence of right ventricular collapse in diastole, a pericardial drain should be inserted.

This patient had a malignant pericardial effusion.

Summary ★★★
Small QRS complexes and widespread T wave changes consistent with a pericardial effusion.

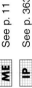

ME See p. 11

IP See p. 363

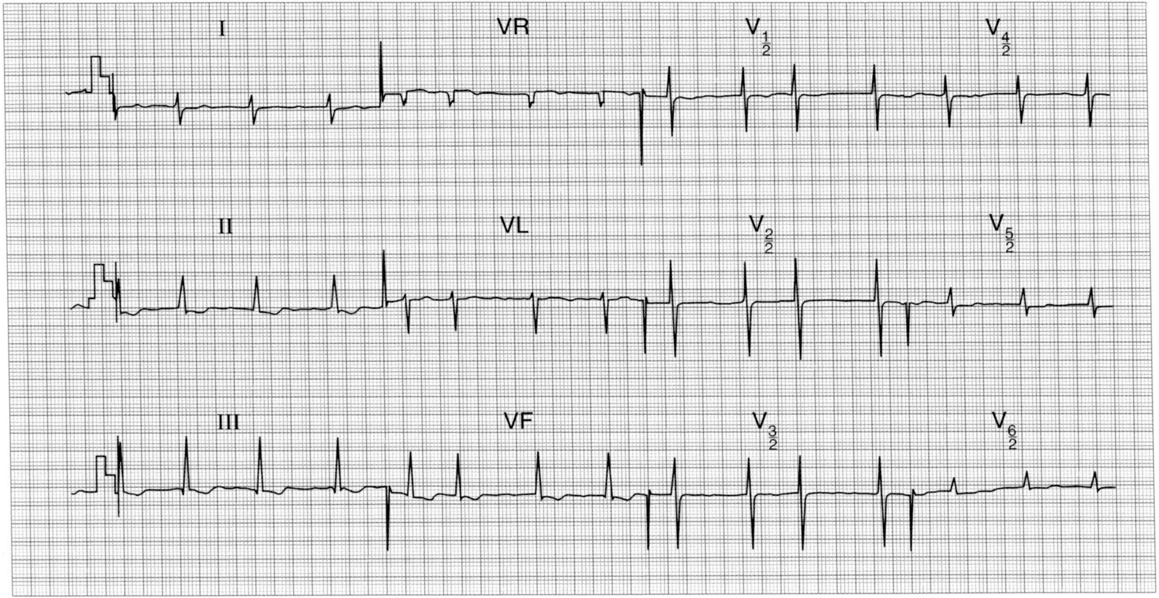

ECG 128 This ECG was recorded from a 65-year-old woman who had had a mitral valve replacement to treat rheumatic valve disease, and who was admitted to hospital with generalised lethargy, nausea and vomiting. What does the ECG show and what would you do? Unfortunately the chemical pathology laboratory burned down last night!

ANSWER 128

The ECG shows (*note*: chest leads at half sensitivity):

- Atrial fibrillation
- Right axis deviation
- Normal QRS complexes, except for a tall R wave in lead V_1
- Generally flattened T waves
- U waves best seen in leads V_4–V_5
- Downward-sloping ST segments, best seen in leads II, III, VF

Clinical interpretation

The atrial fibrillation, and the right axis deviation and tall R waves in lead V_1 (indicating right ventricular hypertrophy) probably pre-date the valve replacement. The flat T waves with obvious U waves suggest hypokalaemia. The downward-sloping ST segments suggest digoxin effect.

What to do

The clinical picture fits hypokalaemia and digoxin toxicity. Since the electrolyte and digoxin levels cannot be measured, stop the patient taking digoxin and any potassium-losing diuretics. Give her potassium orally. Monitoring the T and U waves is a crude but effective way of judging the serum potassium level.

Summary ★★★
Atrial fibrillation, hypokalaemia and digoxin effect.

ME See p. 108

IP See pp. 336 and 366

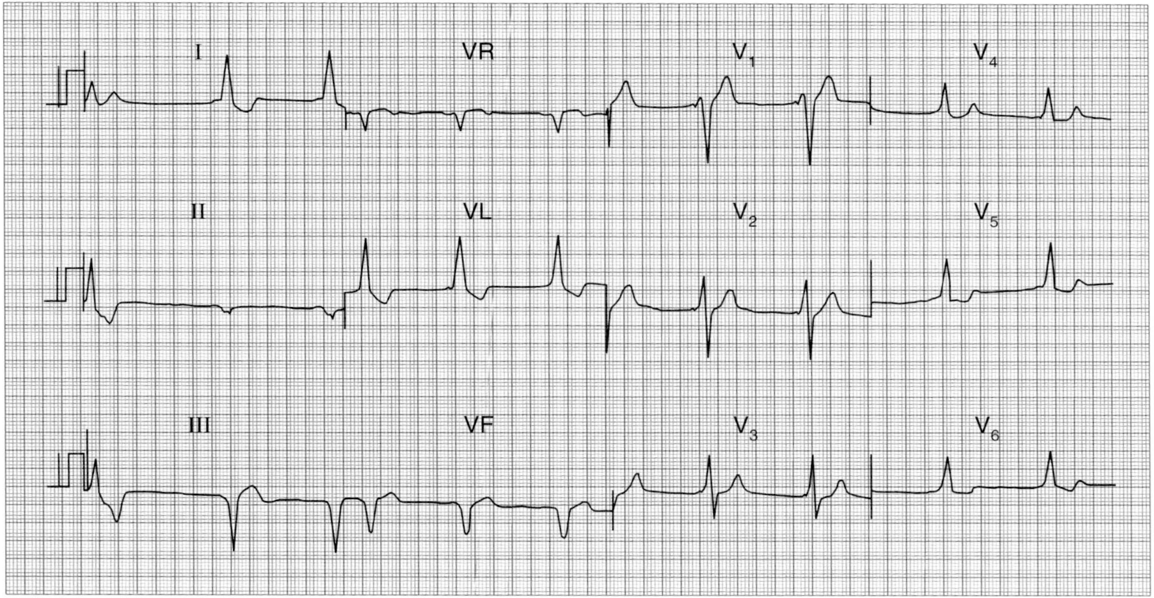

ECG 129 A 20-year-old man is seen in the A & E department with a head injury; there is a vague story of a collapse. What does the ECG show?

ANSWER 129

The ECG shows:

- Sinus rhythm
- Short PR interval
- Left axis deviation
- Broad QRS complexes with a slurred upstroke (delta wave) seen best in leads V_2–V_4
- Inverted T waves in leads I, VL, V_6

Clinical interpretation

The short PR intervals and the delta waves are characteristic of the Wolff–Parkinson–White syndrome. Superficially, leads I, VL and V_6 might mistakenly be interpreted as suggesting left bundle branch block, but it is important to look at all leads because the diagnosis here is best seen in lead V_2.

What to do

The Wolff–Parkinson–White syndrome is associated with paroxysmal tachyarrhythmia, which may cause collapse. Asymptomatic Wolff–Parkinson–White syndrome should be left untreated, but it is important in this case to establish – perhaps by ambulatory ECG recording and exercise testing – whether the patient is having a paroxysmal tachycardia or not.

If there is reason to suppose that an arrhythmia caused a collapse and head injury he needs electrophysiological ablation of the abnormal conducting pathway.

Summary ★★★
Wolff–Parkinson–White syndrome.

ME See p. 81

IP See pp. 37 and 198

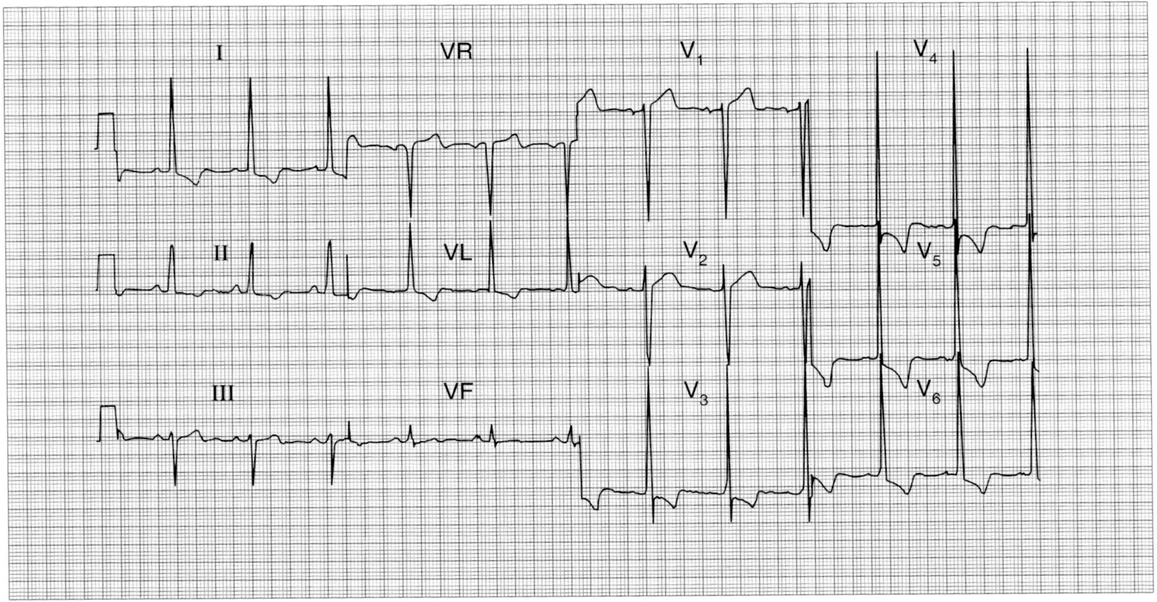

ECG 130 An 85-year-old man is seen in the out-patient department complaining of typical angina and of occasional dizziness when walking up hills. This is his ECG. What is the diagnosis, and what would you do?

ANSWER 130

The ECG shows:

- Sinus rhythm
- Normal axis
- Tall R waves and deep S waves in the chest leads
- Inverted T waves in leads I, II, VL, V_3–V_6

Clinical interpretation

This is marked left ventricular hypertrophy. It can be difficult to distinguish T wave inversion due to ischaemia from the T wave inversion of left ventricular hypertrophy, and when the T wave is inverted in the septal leads (V_3–V_4), ischaemia has to be considered. However, here the change is most marked in the lateral leads, and is associated with 'voltage criteria' for left ventricular hypertrophy. Angina, dizziness and left ventricular hypertrophy in an 85-year-old are almost certainly due to tight aortic stenosis, though hypertension is a possibility.

What to do

Look for the signs of aortic stenosis ('plateau' pulse, narrow pulse pressure, displaced apex beat, aortic ejection systolic murmur) and confirm the valve gradient with echocardiography. In this patient the aortic valve gradient was 95 mmHg indicating severe stenosis of the valve. Angina and dizziness indicate severe disease and a poor prognosis: even at the age of 85 years, aortic valve replacement can be a very successful procedure.

Summary ★

Left ventricular hypertrophy.

ME See pp. 93 and 117

IP See p. 117

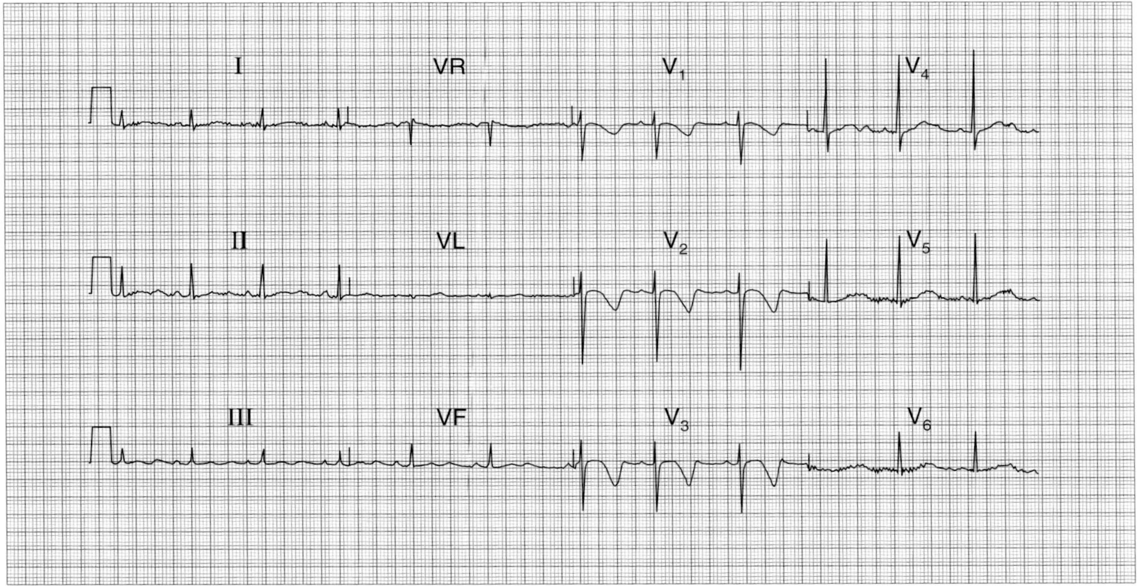

ECG 131 This ECG was recorded from a 15-year-old boy who collapsed while playing football, but was well by the time he was seen. What are the possible diagnoses?

ANSWER 131

The ECG shows:

- Sinus rhythm
- Normal PR and QRS duration
- Normal axis
- Normal QRS complexes
- Inverted T waves in leads V_1–V_3
- Long QT interval (520 ms)

Clinical interpretation

A collapse during exercise raises the possibility of aortic stenosis, hypertrophic cardiomyopathy, or an exercise-induced arrhythmia. This ECG does not show the pattern of left ventricular hypertrophy, so aortic stenosis is unlikely. Anterior T wave inversion is characteristic of hypertrophic cardiomyopathy, but this does not typically cause a prolonged QT interval. Exercise-induced arrhythmias are typical of the familial long-QT syndrome, and this boy's sister had died suddenly.

What to do

Initial treatment is with a beta-blocker, but an ICD (implanted defibrillator) must be considered.

Summary ★★

Congenital long-QT syndrome.

IP See p. 128

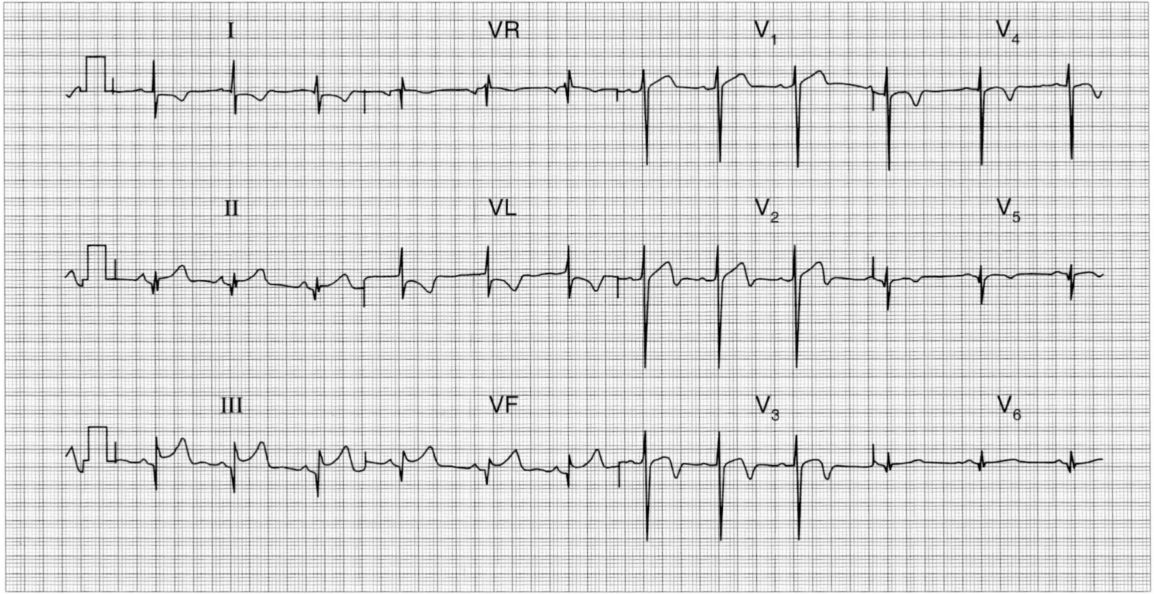

ECG 132 A 70-year-old man, who has had angina for 10 years, is admitted to hospital with severe central chest pain that has been present for 4 h. This is his ECG. What does it show and what would you do?

ANSWER 132

The ECG shows:

- Sinus rhythm
- Normal axis
- Q waves in leads III, VF
- Normal QRS complexes elsewhere
- Raised ST segments in leads II (following small S waves), III, VF
- Biphasic T waves in leads V_2–V_3
- Inverted T waves in leads V_4–V_5

Clinical interpretation

The inferior Q waves suggest an old infarction. The raised ST segments in leads III and VF would be compatible with an acute infarction, though the raised ST segment in lead II is a 'high take-off' because it follows an S wave, and this raises the possibility that the change in leads III and VF may not be significant. The anterior changes suggest a non-Q wave infarction.

What to do

There is enough evidence here to justify thrombolysis which should, of course, be combined with pain relief and aspirin.

Summary ★

Possible old and/or possible new inferior myocardial infarction; non-Q wave anterior myocardial infarction.

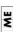

ME See pp. 94 and 103

IP See p. 254

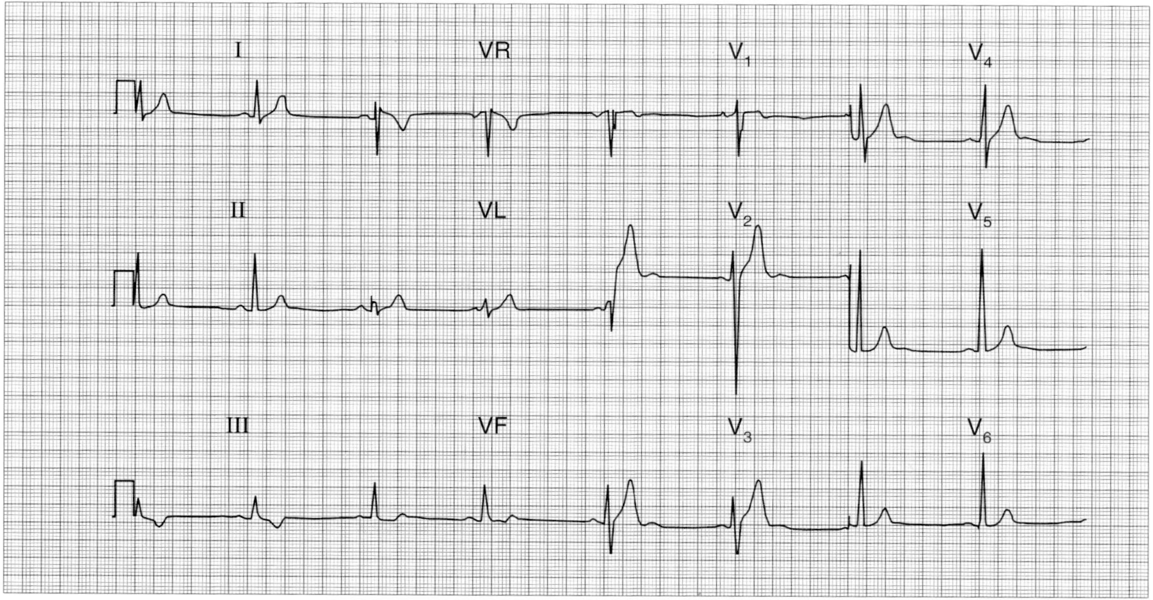

ECG 133 This ECG was recorded from a 30-year-old man as part of a private 'health screening' examination. He was asymptomatic, but is the ECG normal?

ANSWER 133

The ECG shows:

- Sinus rhythm
- Normal axis
- 'Voltage criteria' for left ventricular hypertrophy (height of R wave in lead V_6 plus depth of S wave in lead V_2 exceeds 35 mm)
- Inverted T waves in lead III
- Prominent U waves in leads V_2–V_4

Clinical interpretation

'Voltage criteria' for left ventricular hypertrophy are unreliable, and are often exceeded in young men. There is nothing else here to suggest ventricular hypertrophy. The inverted T waves in lead III are an acceptable variation of normal. When U waves are due to electrolyte abnormalities (usually hypokalaemia), they are associated with flattened T waves. When they follow tall T waves, as here, they are normal.

What to do

Provided the patient's blood pressure is normal and the examination reveals no other cause for left ventricular hypertrophy, such as aortic valve disease, no further action is required.

Summary ★★★

Normal ECG.

IP See pp. 89 and 96

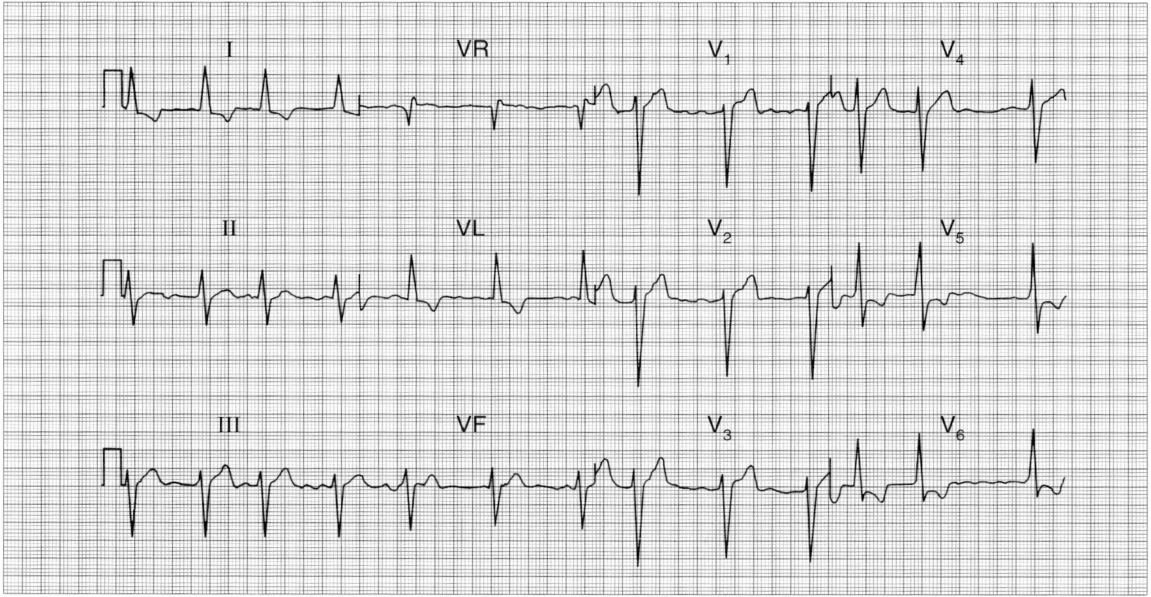

ECG 134 This ECG was recorded from a 60-year-old man admitted to hospital with severe heart failure. What does it show and what would you do?

ANSWER 134

The ECG shows:

- Atrial fibrillation
- Left anterior hemiblock
- Left ventricular hypertrophy by 'voltage criteria' (height of R waves in lead V_6 plus depth of S waves in lead V_1 = 40 mm)
- Lateral T wave inversion

Clinical interpretation

Despite atrial fibrillation, the ventricular rate is well controlled. Left anterior hemiblock indicates disease of the conduction system. The lateral T wave inversion may be due to intraventricular conduction delay, to left ventricular hypertrophy, or may be due to ischaemia. The T wave changes do not have the characteristics of digoxin effect.

What to do

It is essential to know what treatment the patient is already receiving. If he is not taking digoxin this must be used cautiously, because the ventricular rate is slower than one might expect in atrial fibrillation. It is important to seek a cause for left ventricular hypertrophy, remembering that the patient's present blood pressure may not be representative of its usual level.

Summary ★★★

Atrial fibrillation, left anterior hemiblock and probable left ventricular hypertrophy.

ME See pp. 46, 78 and 91

IP See pp. 20 and 320

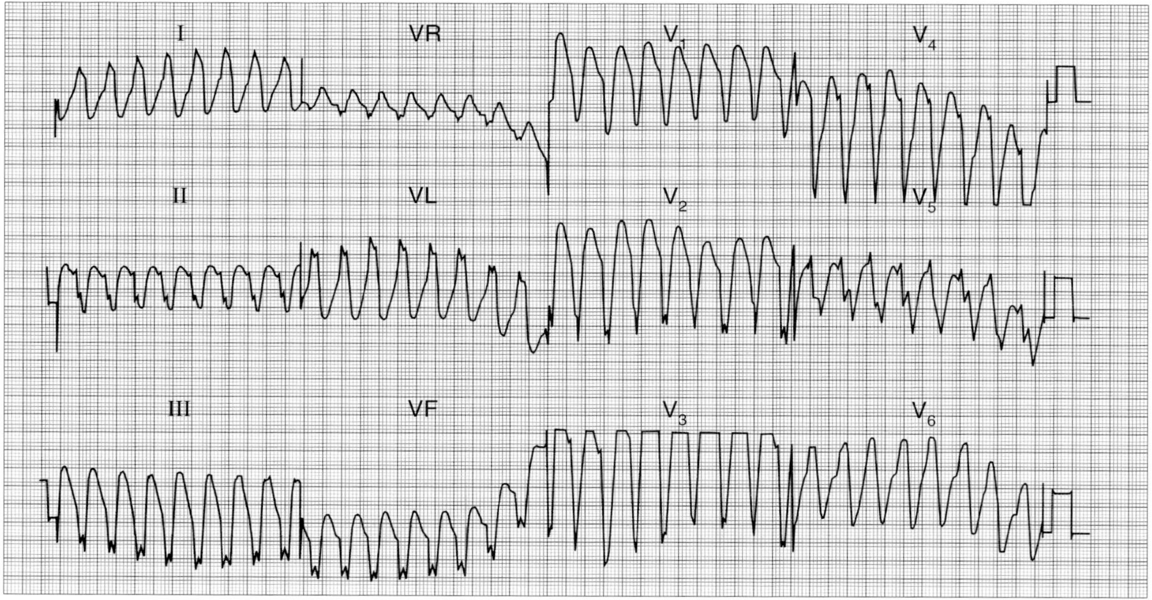

ECG 135 A 60-year-old man had complained of occasional episodes of palpitations for several years. Between attacks he was well, there were no physical abnormalities, and his ECG was normal. Eventually this ECG was recorded during one of his attacks. What is the arrhythmia and what would you do?

ANSWER 135

The ECG shows:

- Regular broad-complex tachycardia
- QRS complex duration 160 ms
- Left axis deviation
- Indeterminate QRS complex configuration, but the complexes point downwards in all the chest leads, with a QS pattern in lead V_6

Clinical interpretation

The combination of broad-complex, regular tachycardia; 'concordant' QRS complexes pointing downwards in all leads; and the QS pattern in lead V_6 is characteristic of ventricular tachycardia.

What to do

Patients who only have occasional episodes of an arrhythmia, and who are otherwise well, are always difficult to manage. This patient should certainly have an echocardiogram to exclude a cardiomyopathy, and an exercise test to exclude ischaemia and exercise-induced arrhythmias. At the age of 60 years, coronary angiography is probably indicated. Treatment with amiodarone is as effective as the selection of an anti-arrhythmic agent on the basis of repeated electrophysiological studies.

If the episodes were causing syncope an implanted defibrillator could be considered.

Summary ★★
Ventricular tachycardia.

ME See p. 75

IP See p. 170

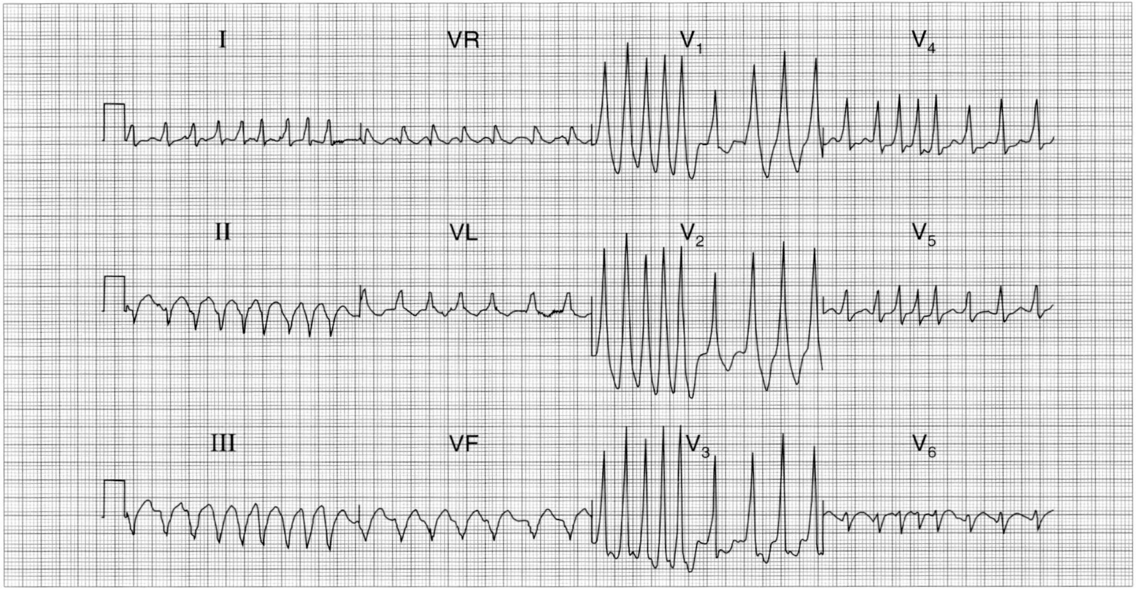

ECG 136 A 25-year-old woman, who had had episodes of what sound like a paroxysmal tachycardia for 10 years, produced this ECG when seen during an attack. What is the rhythm, and what is the underlying problem?

ANSWER 136

The ECG shows:

- Irregular tachycardia at about 200/min
- No consistent P waves visible
- Left axis
- QRS duration varies between about 120 and 160 ms
- QRS shows a dominant R wave in lead V_1 and a prominent S wave in lead V_6
- After the longer pauses, the upstroke of the QRS complexes appear slurred

Clinical interpretation

The marked irregularity of this rhythm must be explained by atrial fibrillation. The broad QRS complexes might be due to right bundle branch block, but the dominant R wave in lead V_1, together with the slurred upstroke of the QRS complex in at least some leads, indicate a Wolff–Parkinson–White syndrome (type A).

What to do

The combination of a Wolff–Parkinson–White syndrome and atrial fibrillation is very dangerous, for it can degenerate to ventricular fibrillation. The arrhythmia needs treating as an emergency whatever the clinical state of the patient. It is important not to use drugs that may block the atrioventricular node and increase conduction through the accessory pathway, for this will increase the risk of ventricular fibrillation. Therefore, adenosine, digoxin, verapamil and lignocaine are contraindicated. The drugs that slow conduction in the accessory pathway, and are therefore safe, are the beta-blockers, flecainide and amiodarone. Thereafter, an electrophysiological study to identify and ablate the accessory pathway is essential.

Summary ★★★

Atrial fibrillation and a Wolff–Parkinson–White syndrome.

ME See pp. 78 and 81

IP See p. 198

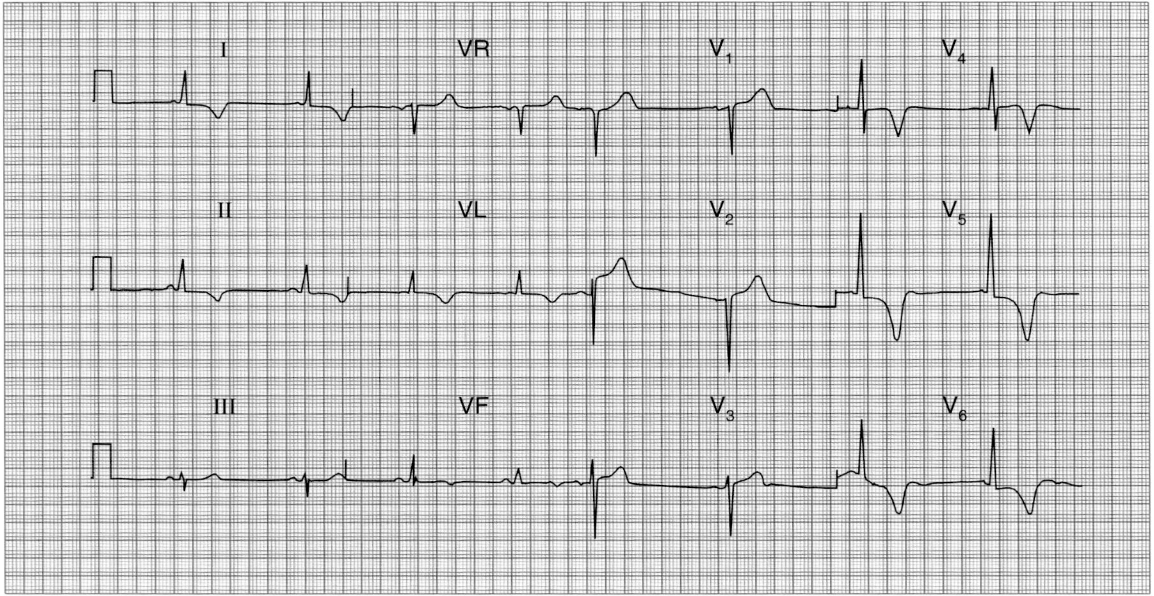

ECG 137 A 35-year-old white man is seen in the out-patient department complaining of chest pain on exertion, sometimes with exertion-induced dizziness, and this is his ECG. What is the likely diagnosis? What physical signs would you look for?

ANSWER 137

The ECG shows:

- Sinus rhythm
- Normal axis
- Normal QRS complexes
- Marked T wave inversion in leads I, II, VL, V_4–V_6

Clinical interpretation

Anterolateral T wave inversion as gross as this may be due to a non-Q wave infarction, or even to left ventricular hypertrophy. However, there are no other features of left ventricular hypertrophy on this trace, which is fairly characteristic of hypertrophic cardiomyopathy.

What to do

Physical signs of hypertrophic cardiomyopathy include a 'jerky pulse'; an aortic flow murmur which is characteristically louder after the pause that follows an extrasystole; and mitral regurgitation. Hypertrophic cardiomyopathy is best diagnosed by echocardiography, which will show asymmetric septal hypertrophy, systolic anterior movement of the mitral valve apparatus, and sometimes early closure of the aortic valve.

This patient's echocardiogram showed all these features confirming the diagnosis of hypertrophic cardiomyopathy.

Summary ★★★
Gross T wave inversion in the anterolateral leads, suggesting hypertrophic cardiomyopathy.

IP See p. 328

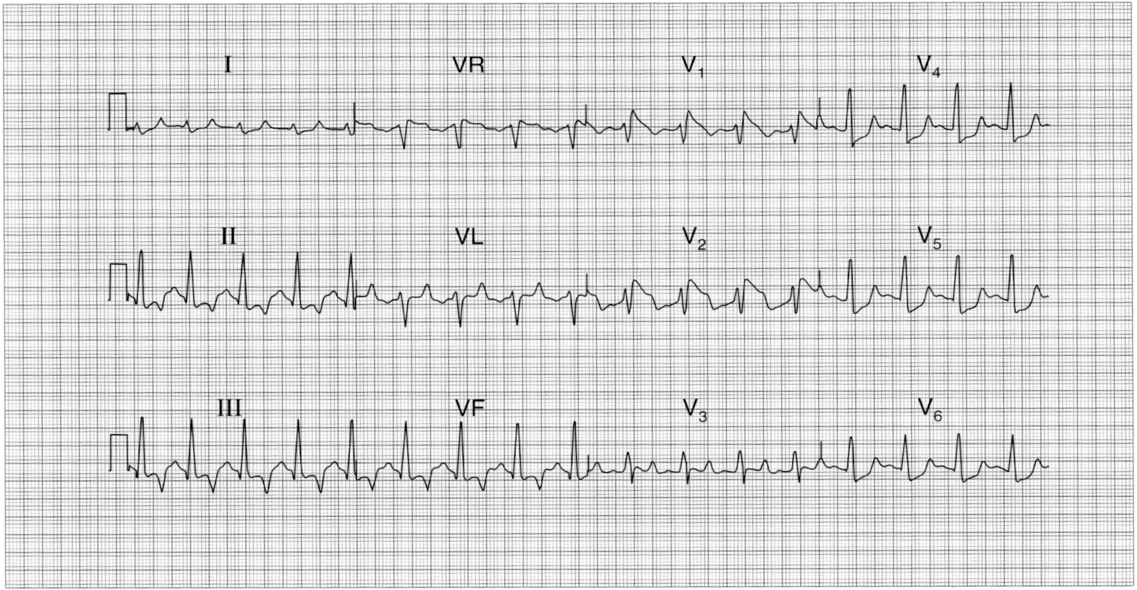

ECG 138 This ECG was recorded from a 30-year-old woman admitted with diabetic ketoacidosis. Any comments?

ANSWER 138

The ECG shows:

- Sinus rhythm
- Normal PR interval
- Normal axis
- QRS duration upper limit of normal of 120 ms, but QRS complexes otherwise normal
- ST segment not easy to identify, but appears raised in leads V_1 and V_2, and depressed (upward-sloping) in leads V_4–V_6
- T waves inverted in the inferior leads, and peaked in all leads

Clinical interpretation

These changes are characteristic of hyperkalaemia, which of course is likely to be present in diabetic ketoacidosis.

What to do

This ECG should alert you to check the serum potassium level immediately: in this patient it was found to be 7.1 mmol/l. It settled rapidly with treatment of the diabetes.

Summary ★★★
Hyperkalaemia.

ME See p. 108
IP See p. 366

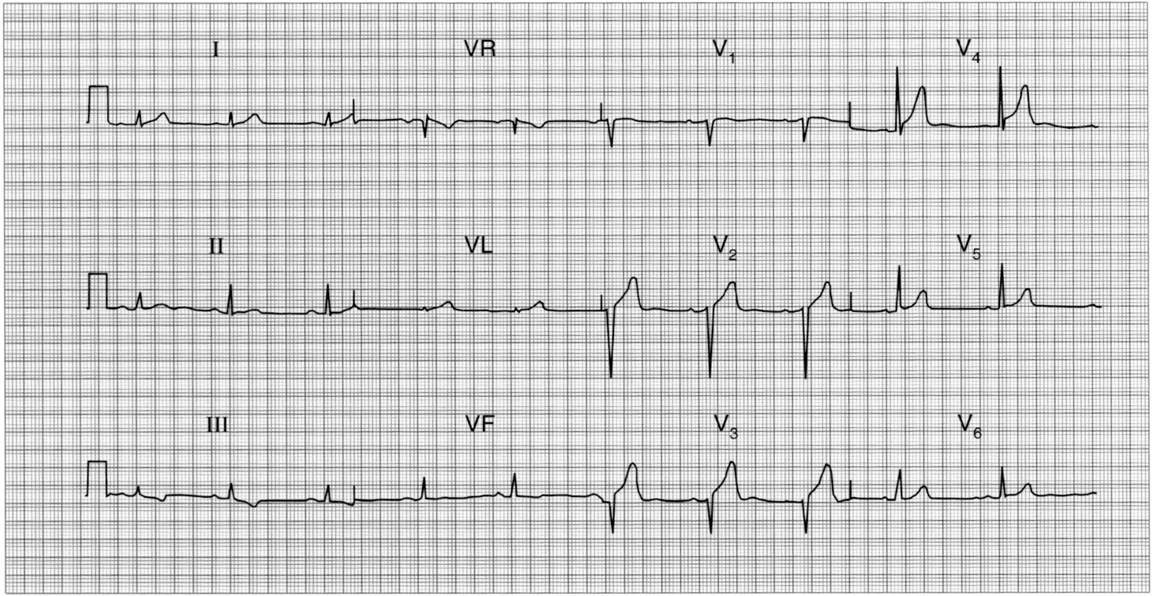

ECG 139 This ECG was recorded as part of the health screening of an asymptomatic 40-year-old man. How would you proceed?

ANSWER 139

The ECG shows:

- Sinus rhythm
- Normal axis
- Loss of R waves in lead V_3
- 'High take-off' ST segments in lead V_4
- Inverted T waves in leads III, VF

Clinical interpretation

A loss of R waves in lead V_3, with the sudden appearance of the R wave in lead V_4, could indicate an old anterior infarct. The raised ST segments in lead V_4, following S waves, are certainly a normal variant. The T wave inversion in the inferior leads is probably 'non-specific', but could be due to ischaemia.

What to do

With a totally asymptomatic patient it is very difficult to know how to interpret this ECG. The likelihood is that the changes are all non-specific, but ischaemia cannot be excluded on this record. It would be worth repeating the ECG to see if the loss of R waves in lead V_3 results from faulty positioning of the chest electrodes when this ECG was recorded. It would also be worth asking the patient to take a deep breath when the inferior leads are recorded, to see if the T waves normalize. If the ECG continues to show the changes seen here, an exercise test is the only way forward.

Summary ★★★
Probably normal with 'high take-off' ST segments, but possible inferior ischaemia and possible old anterior infarction.

IP See p. 51

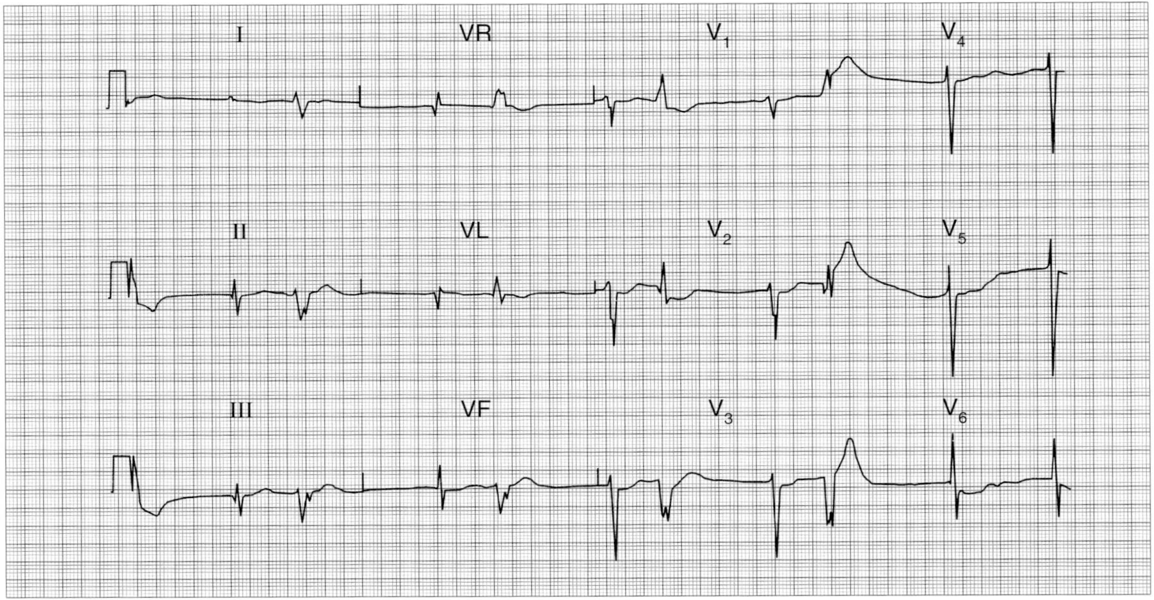

ECG 140 A 60-year-old woman, with long-standing heart failure of uncertain cause, complains of anorexia, weight loss, and general weakness and lethargy. Does this ECG help with her diagnosis and management?

ANSWER 140

The ECG shows:

- Atrial fibrillation
- Coupled ventricular extrasystoles
- Q waves in lead VL (in the supraventricular beats)
- Flattened T waves and prominent U waves (best seen in lead V_3)
- Sloping ST segment depression in lead V_6

Clinical interpretation

A patient with heart failure who is in atrial fibrillation will probably be receiving digoxin and diuretics. The history of anorexia and weight loss suggests digoxin toxicity and the weakness could be due to hypokalaemia. The ECG supports this. Lead V_6 shows digoxin effect, and coupled ventricular extrasystoles are a feature of digoxin toxicity. The flat T waves and prominent U waves suggest hypokalaemia.

What to do

Remember that hypokalaemia potentiates the effect of digoxin. Therefore stop the digoxin, check the electrolytes, and give oral potassium supplements. Do not give antiarrhythmic agents. Treat the heart failure with vasodilators.

This woman improved dramatically when her digoxin dose was reduced, she was given oral potassium, and then she was started on an angiotensin-converting enzyme inhibitor and a reduced dose of diuretics.

Summary ★★★

Atrial fibrillation with ventricular extrasystoles; probable digoxin toxicity and hypokalaemia.

ME See pp. 78 and 107

IP See pp. 368 and 372

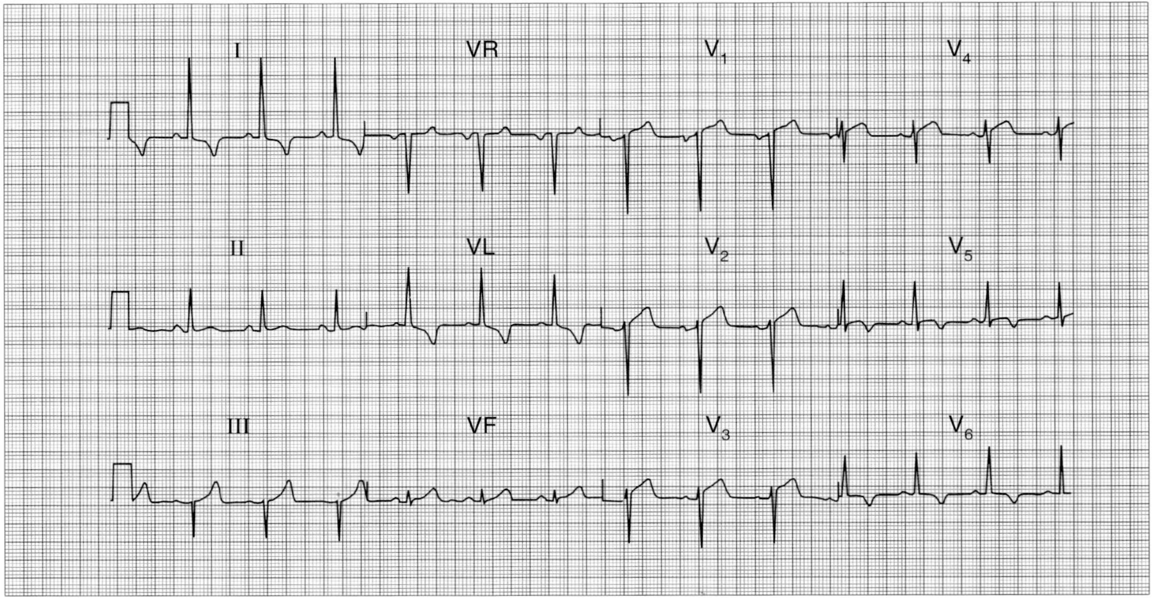

ECG 141 A 50-year-old man complains of typical angina. His blood pressure is 150/90, and he has an aortic ejection systolic murmur. This is his ECG. What is the probable cause of his angina, and what would you do?

ANSWER 141

The ECG shows:

- Sinus rhythm
- Normal axis
- Normal QRS complexes
- Raised ST segments following S waves in leads V_4–V_5
- Inverted T waves in leads I, VL, V_5–V_6

Clinical interpretation

The raised ST segments in leads V_4–V_5 are due to 'high take-off' and are not important. The lateral T wave inversion could indicate left ventricular hypertrophy or ischaemia, and this patient could have aortic stenosis or coronary disease. In the absence of tall R waves, lateral ischaemia seems more likely than left ventricular hypertrophy, but it is often difficult to distinguish between these on the ECG.

What to do

Echocardiography will show whether the patient has significant aortic valve disease. Remember that anaemia can cause systolic murmurs and angina, though probably not this degree of T wave inversion.

This patient had coronary disease.

Summary ★★★
Probable lateral ischaemia, but possible left ventricular hypertrophy.

ME See pp. 93 and 103
IP See pp. 302 and 324

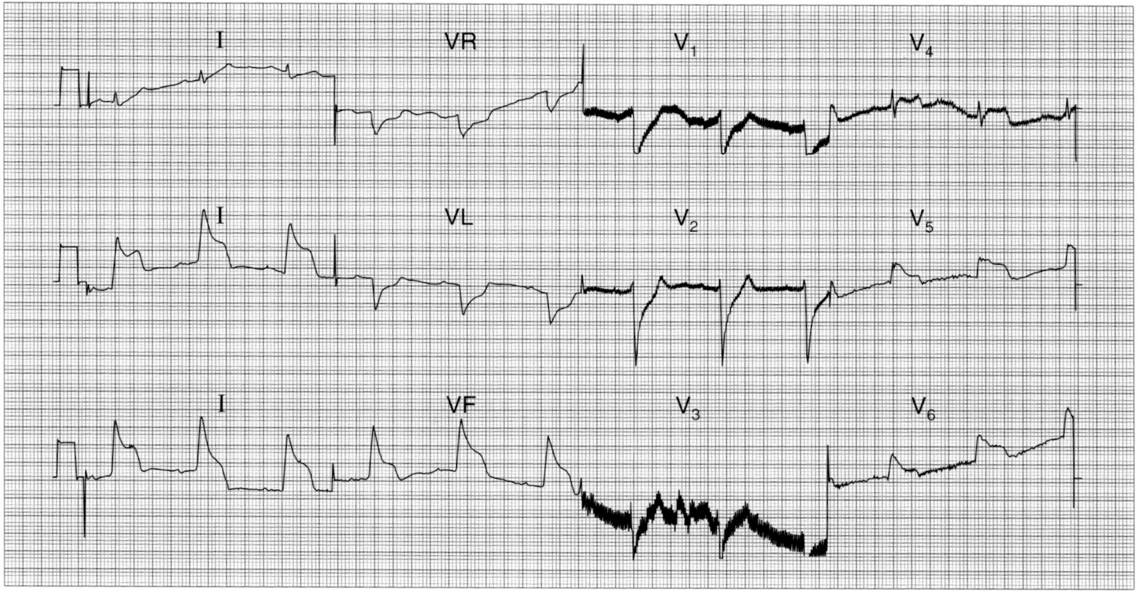

ECG 142 This ECG was recorded by paramedics from a 50-year-old woman who had had episodes of chest pain for several years, but who called an ambulance because of a severe attack. By the time she reached the A & E department her pain had gone, and her ECG was found to be totally normal. What has happened?

ANSWER 142

The ECG shows:

- Artefacts in leads V_1 and V_3
- Sinus rhythm
- Normal PR interval
- Normal axis
- Broad QRS complexes (about 160 ms)
- Raised ST segments in leads II, III, VF, V_4–V_6
- T waves probably normal

Clinical interpretation

These appearances seem to indicate an acute inferolateral myocardial infarction. An alternative explanation, given the widespread changes, would be pericarditis. However, since the ECG reverted to normal when the pain cleared it seems likely that they represent Prinzmetal's variant angina.

What to do

Prinzmetal's variant angina was first described in 1959. It occurs at rest, and the characteristic raised ST segments seen in the ECG are not reproduced by exertion. It has been shown by angiography during pain to be due to spasm of one or more coronary arteries. However, relatively few patients with this type of angina have totally normal arteries, and spasm may occur at the site of atheromatous plaques. Coronary angiography is indicated.

Summary ★★★
Prinzmetal's variant angina.

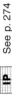

IP See p. 274

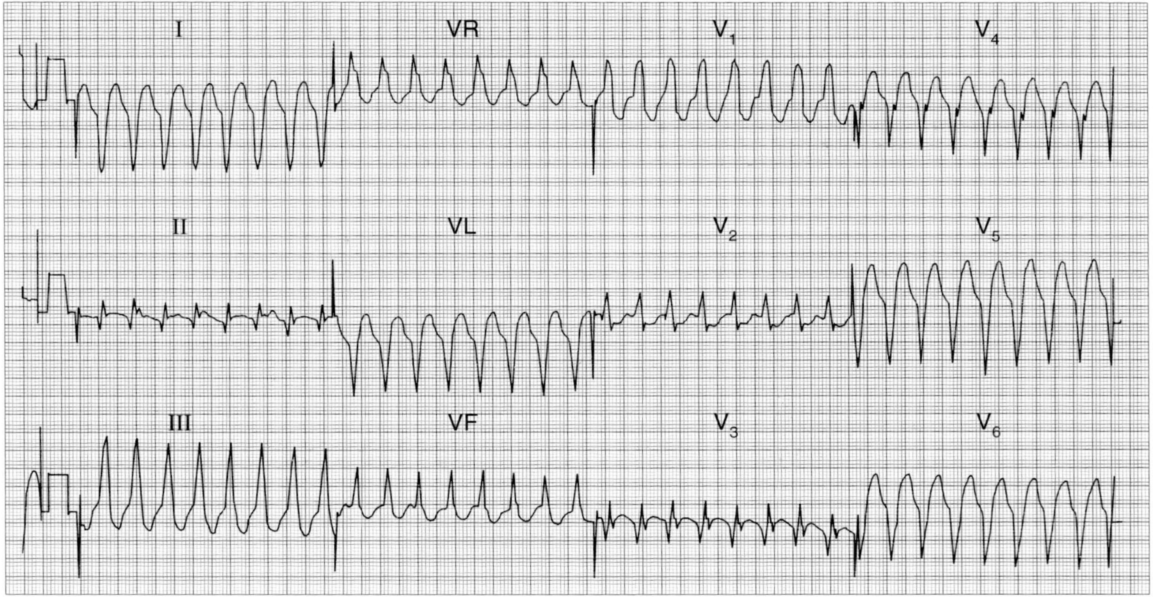

ECG 143 A 45-year-old man was admitted to hospital with a history of 2 h of ischaemic chest pain. His blood pressure was 150/80, and there were no signs of heart failure. What does his ECG show, and how would you treat him?

ANSWER 143

The ECG shows:

- Broad-complex tachycardia, rate 200/min
- No P waves
- Right axis deviation
- QRS complex duration about 140 ms
- Right bundle branch block pattern, with the R peak taller than the R^1 peak in lead V_1
- Non-concordant QRS complexes with negative QS pattern in lead V_6 (i.e. complexes are upwards in lead V_1 but downwards in lead V_6)

Clinical interpretation

This is either ventricular tachycardia or supraventricular tachycardia with right bundle branch block. In favour of the former are the relatively wide QRS complexes and the fact that the R peak is greater than the R^1 peak in lead V_1 (i.e. this is not the typical right bundle branch block pattern). Against ventricular tachycardia are the right axis deviation and the different directions of the QRS complexes in the chest leads.

What to do

The problem is to decide whether the patient had a myocardial infarction complicated by ventricular tachycardia, or whether the arrhythmia is causing the anginal pain. Since he is haemodynamically stable he needs pain relief, carotid sinus pressure, intravenous adenosine and intravenous lignocaine in that order. If in doubt, or if his blood pressure were to fall or he were to develop heart failure, the safest course of action would be DC cardioversion.

This patient needed cardioversion and the ECG then showed an anterior infarction. The rhythm was probably ventricular tachycardia.

Summary ★★★
Broad-complex tachycardia of uncertain origin.

ME See p. 77

IP See pp. 170 and 393

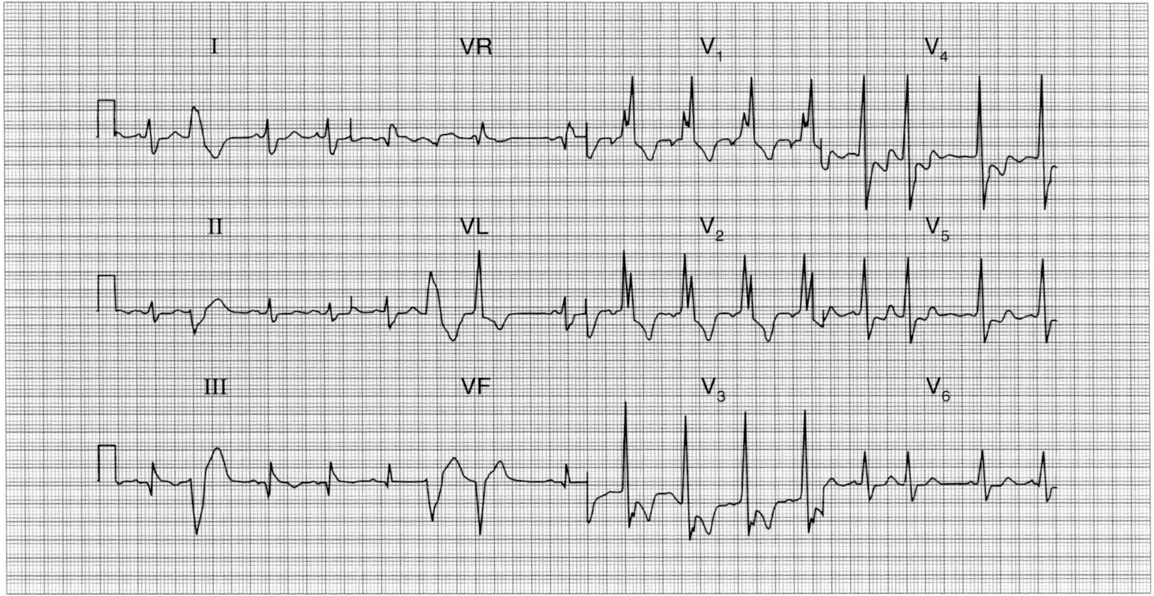

ECG 144 This ECG was recorded from a 65-year-old man who complained of breathlessness and who showed the physical signs of moderate heart failure. What does this ECG show? Does it have implications for treatment?

ANSWER 144

The ECG shows:

- Sinus rhythm
- Multifocal ventricular extrasystoles
- Right bundle branch block
- Q waves in the sinus beats in leads III, VF

Clinical interpretation

The presence of Q waves in the inferior leads suggests an old infarction. Ischaemic disease is therefore probably the cause of the extrasystoles and the right bundle branch block.

What to do

Control of the heart failure may well cause the extrasystoles to disappear; the extrasystoles should not be treated with antiarrhythmic drugs. The presence of multifocal extrasystoles should alert you to consider electrolyte abnormalities and digoxin toxicity.

Summary ★★

Multifocal ventricular extrasystoles, right bundle branch block, and probable old inferior myocardial infarction.

ME See pp. 36, 64 and 103

IP See p. 259

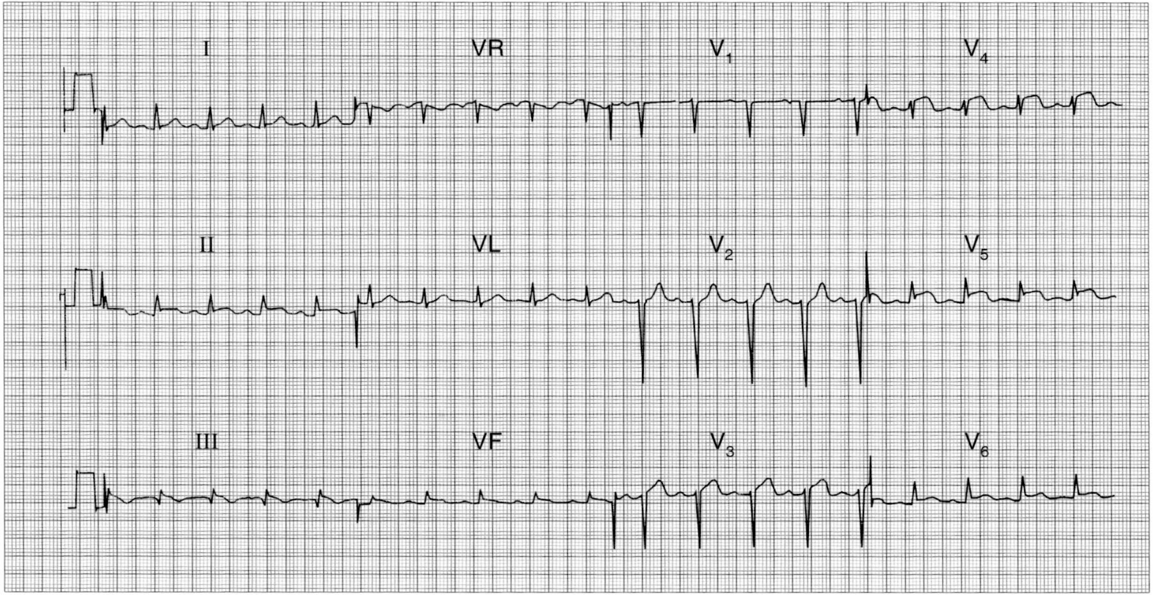

ECG 145 This ECG was recorded in the A & E department from a 25-year-old man with severe chest pain. No physical abnormalities had been detected, but having seen the ECG what would you look for and what would you do?

ANSWER 145

The ECG shows:

- Sinus rhythm
- Normal axis
- Normal QRS complexes
- Raised ST segments in leads I, II, III, VF, V_4–V_6

Clinical interpretation

The raised ST segments in leads I and V_4 follow S waves and are therefore 'high take-off' and are of no significance. The ST elevation elsewhere could indicate an acute infarction, but since the change is so widespread, pericarditis seems more probable.

What to do

In a 25-year-old, pericarditis is a much more likely diagnosis than infarction and thrombolysis must be avoided. The diagnosis is made by lying the patient flat, when a pericardial rub will become much easier to hear. Echocardiography will show a pericardial effusion if one is present.

Summary ★★★
Widespread ST segment elevation, suggesting pericarditis.

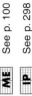

ME See p. 100

IP See p. 298

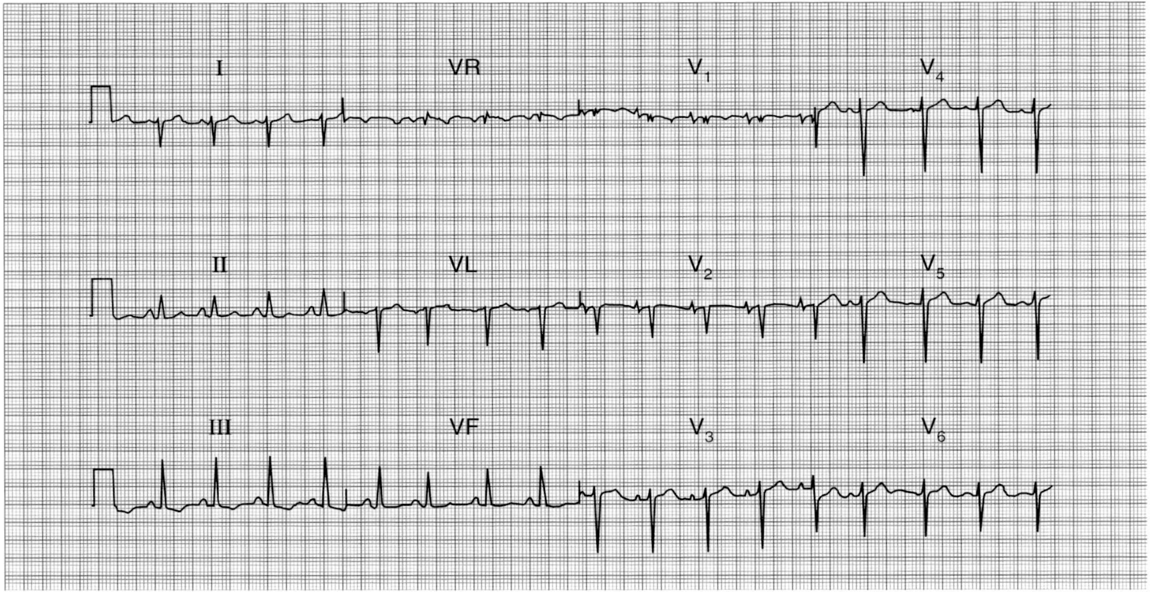

ECG 146 This ECG was recorded from a 70-year-old man who complained of breathlessness. What abnormalities does it show and what is the most likely diagnosis?

ANSWER 146

The ECG shows:

- Sinus rhythm
- Peaked P waves, best seen in leads V_1–V_2
- Right axis deviation (deep S waves in lead I)
- RSR pattern with normal QRS duration in lead V_1 (partial right bundle branch block)
- Deep S waves in lead V_6, with no left ventricular pattern

Clinical interpretation
Peaked P waves suggest right atrial hypertrophy. The partial right bundle branch block pattern is not significant. Right axis deviation may be seen in tall thin people with normal hearts, but with the deep S waves in lead V_6 it suggests right ventricular hypertrophy. A lack of development of a left ventricular pattern in the V leads (i.e. deep S waves persisting into lead V_6) results from the right ventricle occupying most of the pericardium. This is sometimes called 'clockwise rotation' (looking at the heart from below) and is characteristic of chronic lung disease.

What to do
A chest X-ray examination, including a lateral view (which shows the right ventricle better), and lung function tests will be more helpful than echocardiography.

Summary ★★
Right atrial hypertrophy and probable chronic lung disease.

ME See pp. 89 and 91

IP See p. 342

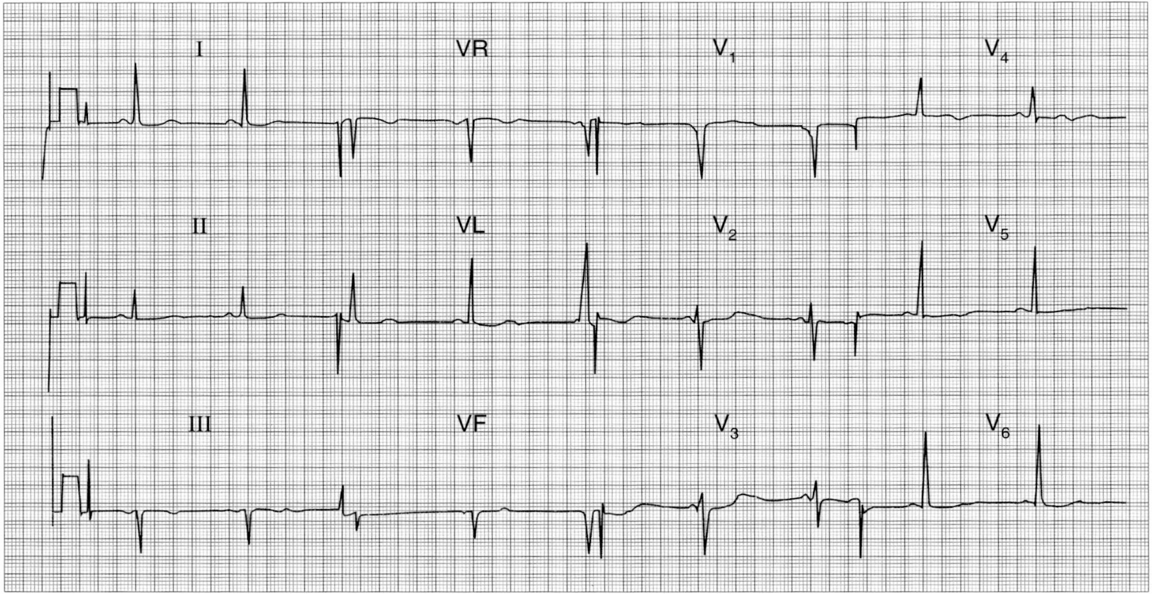

ECG 147 This ECG was recorded from a 15-year-old boy who collapsed while playing football. His brother had died suddenly. What does the ECG show and what clinical possibilities should be considered?

ANSWER 147

The ECG shows:

- Sinus rhythm
- Normal PR intervals except for the third complex in lead VL, where there is a suggestion of pre-excitation
- Normal axis
- Normal QRS complexes
- Prolonged QT intervals (about 640 ms)
- Prominent U waves, best seen in the chest leads

Clinical interpretation

The most important abnormalities here are the prolonged QT intervals and the presence of U waves. This is a pattern often associated with ventricular tachycardia of the 'torsade' type and with sudden death.

What to do

The family history suggests that this may well be an example of one of the congenital forms of prolonged QT interval – the Jervell–Lange–Nielson or the Romano–Ward syndrome. These are characterized by episodes of loss of consciousness in children, often at times of increased sympathetic nervous system activity, and beta-blockers are the immediate form of treatment. The insertion of a permanent defibrillator may be necessary. Prolonged QT interval syndrome is also associated with antiarrhythmic drugs (quinidine, procainamide, disopyramide, amiodarone and sotalol) and with other drugs such as ketanserin, prenylamine, the tricyclic antidepressants, erythromycin, thioridazine and lidoflazine. Electrolyte abnormalities (low potassium, magnesium or calcium levels) also prolong the QT interval.

Summary ★★★
Marked prolongation of the QT interval with pathological U waves – the 'long QT' syndrome.

IP See p. 128

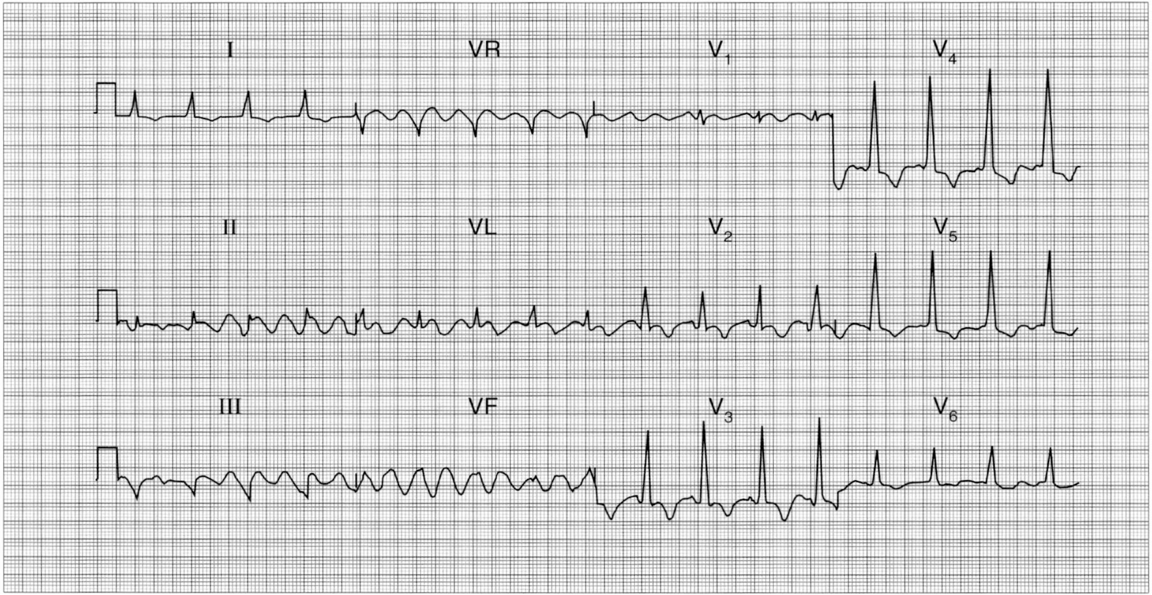

ECG 148 The houseofficer from the health care of the elderly ward is puzzled by this ECG and asks for your help. What questions would you ask him?

ANSWER 148

The ECG shows:

- Sinus rhythm
- Slow rhythmic waves, the baseline in some ways resembling atrial flutter, but slower and coarser
- Short PR intervals
- Slurred upstroke of the QRS complexes, particularly in lead I
- T wave inversion in the anterior leads

Clinical interpretation

The slow rhythmic variation is due to muscle tremor, and is not cardiac in origin. The short PR intervals, slurred upstroke of the QRS complexes and inverted T waves are due to the Wolff–Parkinson–White syndrome.

What to do

Ask if the patient has Parkinson's disease: a Parkinsonian tremor would explain the baseline variation. Does the patient give a history of palpitations or syncope? This would be the only significant problem that the Wolff–Parkinson–White syndrome might cause in an elderly patient.

Summary ★★★

Muscle artefact, possibly Parkinson's disease; Wolff–Parkinson–White syndrome.

IP See pp. 104 and 357

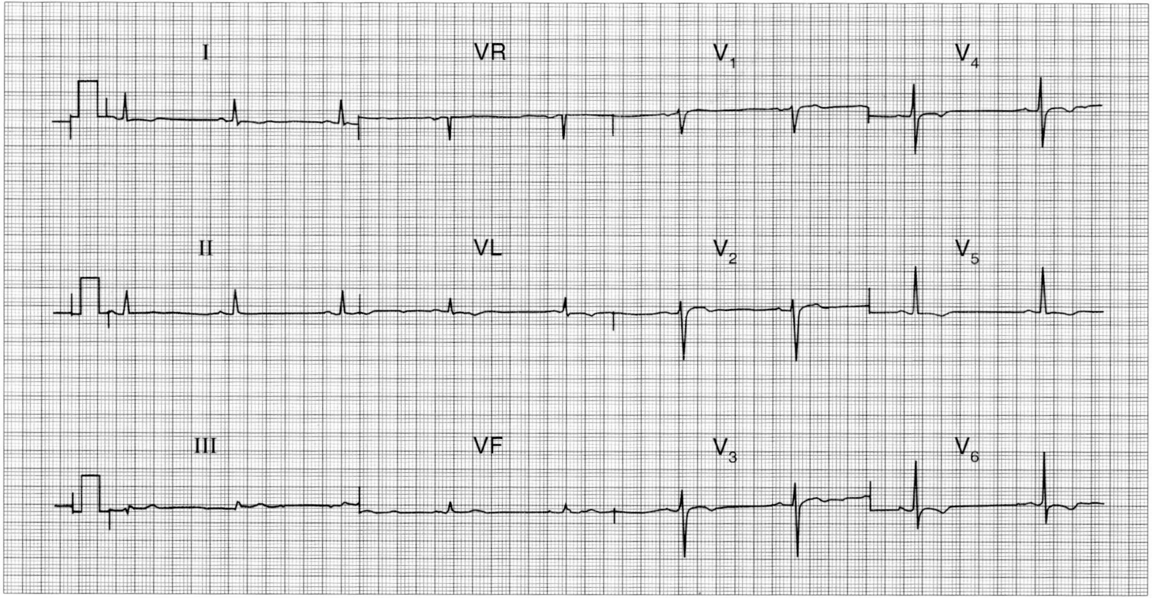

ECG 149 A 30-year-old woman, who had been treated for depression for several years, was admitted to hospital as an emergency following deliberate self-harm involving a small number of aspirin tablets. There were no abnormalities on examination but this was her ECG. Does it worry you?

ANSWER 149

The ECG shows:

- Sinus rhythm
- Normal axis
- Normal QRS complexes
- T wave inversion in leads I, VL, V_4–V_6

Clinical interpretation

Anterolateral T wave inversion is most commonly due to ischaemia, but this seems unlikely in a young woman with no evidence of heart disease. A cardiomyopathy would be another possibility, but repolarization (T wave) abnormalities can be caused by lithium therapy.

What to do

As always when a diagnosis is not clear, find out what drugs the patient is taking. This patient was taking lithium, and exercise testing and echocardiography showed no evidence of heart disease.

Summary ★★★
Anterolateral T wave inversion due to lithium therapy.

IP See p. 372

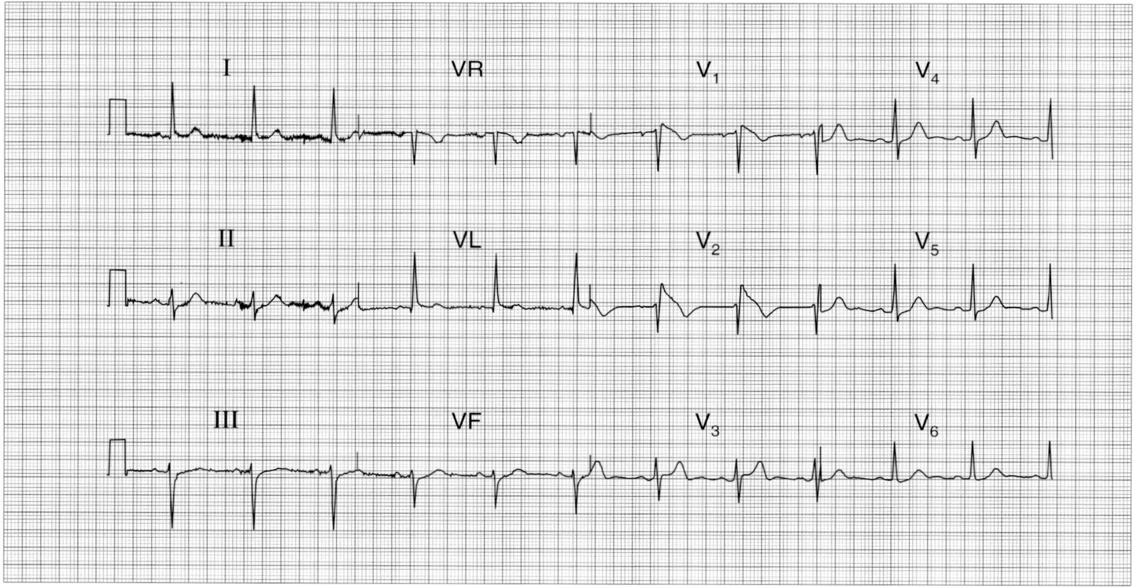

ECG 150 This ECG was recorded from a 40-year-old man who was admitted after collapsing in a supermarket. By the time he was seen he was well, and there were no abnormal physical signs. Would you pass this ECG as normal?

ANSWER 150

The ECG shows:

- Sinus rhythm, rate 70/min
- Normal PR and QRS duration
- Normal axis
- QRS complexes in leads V_1–V_2 show an RSR pattern
- ST segment elevated, and downward-sloping, in V_1–V_2
- Normal T waves

Clinical interpretation

This is not a normal ECG. The appearances in leads V_1 and V_2 are characteristic of the Brugada syndrome.

What to do

The Brugada syndrome involves a genetic abnormality that alters sodium transport in the myocardium, and predisposes to ventricular tachycardia and fibrillation. This patient's collapse may well have been due to an arrhythmia. The syndrome is often familial. The ECG changes are not constant, and on the day after admission this patient's ECG was perfectly normal. The ECG changes can be induced, and ventricular tachycardia caused, by antiarrhythmic drugs. The only treatment is an implanted defibrillator.

Summary ★★★
Brugada syndrome.

IP See p. 134

Index

Note: Numbers refer to page numbers not question numbers; numbers in *italics* refer to pages showing ECG traces